RAW LIVING

DETOX YOUR LIFE AND EAT THE HIGH ENERGY WAY

Kate Wood

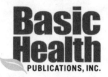

Basic Health
PUBLICATIONS, INC.

The information contained in this book is based upon the research and personal and professional experiences of the author. It is not intended as a substitute for consulting with your physician or other healthcare provider. Any attempt to diagnose and treat an illness should be done under the direction of a healthcare professional.

The publisher does not advocate the use of any particular healthcare protocol but believes the information in this book should be available to the public. The publisher and author are not responsible for any adverse effects or consequences resulting from the use of the suggestions, preparations, or procedures discussed in this book. Should the reader have any questions concerning the appropriateness of any procedures or preparation mentioned, the author and the publisher strongly suggest consulting a professional healthcare advisor.

Basic Health Publications, Inc.
28812 Top of the World Drive
Laguna Beach, CA 92651
949-715-7327 • www.basichealthpub.com

Library of Congress Cataloging-in-Publication Data
Wood, Kate.
    Raw living : detox your life and eat the high-energy way / Kate Wood.
        p. cm.
    "Originally published by Published by Grub Street, 4 Rainham Close, London."
    ISBN 978-1-59120-253-0
1. Raw food diet. I. Title.

    RM237.5.W66   2008
    613.2'6—dc22

                                        2008037373

In-house Editor: Tara Durkin
Typesetting/Book design: Gary A. Rosenberg
Cover design: Mike Stromberg

Printed in the United States of America

10   9   8   7   6   5   4   3   2   1

Contents

THE RECIPES

To Chris, Reuben, Ethan,
Zachary, Alxxx, Shazzie, Evie, and Dani,
for loving me enough to let me have my cake and eat it.

Foreword

When Kate Wood's first book, *Eat Smart Eat Raw,* came out, I was so excited! Kate's book was so practical, I actually used the recipes. What a revelation for me! Now, after seeing the recipes in her second book, I am so glad that Kate has done it again.

I have a confession to make. Over the past year, I've been eating Kate's food at every opportunity. OK, I have a further confession to make, I haven't been making her recipes, she has! I've been loitering in her large sofa'd up kitchen and marveling at the way she just presents me with a bowl, a smile, and a question such as, "Would you like some spinach cakes?" I enjoy the spinach cakes, I enjoy the company, and then I'm presented with a delicious pudding and the same smile as before. Her eldest son, Reuben, does the same, "I've made some sweet corn and almond soup. Would you like some?" Then he gently warms it and hands me a bowl, topped with crunchy bits. My daughter Evie wanders over to the dehydrator, which is always on, always making something. "I want a cookie!" She demands. Kate produces tomato chips, cookies, and flapjacks for Evie to enjoy.

This is the essence of *Raw Living.* It's not just a collection of raw ingredients thrown together haphazardly. It's a raw family's gift destined to help us all create wonderful food choices for our families.

Raw Living is for everyone! We all know we need more fruit, vegetables, and raw foods in our diet. So many more of us are now listening to the cues that our bodies are giving us: "Be gentle with me, nourish me, love me, give me fresh air, snuggles, and love, and I'll give you the best life ever." We're all waking up to the fact that lighter living in all ways is the only way that makes sense. No nutritionist ever said, "Eat more burgers and fries!" *Raw Living* offers us so many ways in which to nourish ourselves that our bodies can cross it off its list of things to remind us to do.

Kate is the mother of three raw home-schooled boys. She's an author of two books. She's a company director, she has a shop and a cafe. She also likes to party! She manages to do all this because the foods she eats give her the energy to do it. *Raw Living* is an infinite energy bank! Kate is a true example of a superbeing, and you can be too, just by eating her food. OK, you may not get to hang out in her kitchen, but you can eat *Raw Living*'s recipes—it's surely the next best thing!

Kate is also one of the leading lights in the raw chocolate revolution. She's created more delicious chocolates, cakes, cookies, and savory dishes than anyone else I know. Some of them are in this book, so if you can't reach her shop, you can still experience them. Aren't you lucky?

So without further ado, all that remains to be said is: "Let them eat, Kate!"

—Shazzie
Author and Managing Director
of Rawcreation Ltd.

Introduction

*H*ealthy eating is officially "here." It seems you can't move these days for nutritionists advising you what to eat, celebrities endorsing a new diet regimen, governments issuing strategies, or the media supplying alarming statistics. We are becoming a nation of people who take our health seriously, who want to eat the right things, who want to be slim, fit, and youthful. We are realizing that in some foods quality has deteriorated over the past fifty years, to the point where we can no longer get all the nutrients we need from it. And there are so many more stresses to contend with, which deplete our reserves: environmentally in the form of pollution, chemicals in the home, and electromagnetic radiation; and socially, in the fast-paced, high-pressured lives so many of us live these days. If we do not look after ourselves properly, inevitably we become prey to one of the numerous symptoms of ill-health that affect us all—from general fatigue and muddle-headedness, through to asthma, eczema, and psoriasis, all the way to cancer, heart disease, and diabetes.

But it can be very hard to bridge that gap between our good intentions and our day-to-day realities. You may have read half a dozen times now that you need to get lots of essential fatty acids (EFAs) to help prevent depression, but you're still not really sure what to do with that bottle of flax oil at the back of your fridge. You've realized your children's diet is low in minerals, but how do you get them to eat their greens? You're ready to kick the dairy milk habit, but what are you going to replace it with? Or you may simply not have the time and energy to research thoroughly the new foods you should be eating to achieve vitality. That's where *Raw Living* steps in.

1

If you examine all the various nutritional theories and diet plans closely, all that advice has a lot in common. Jill says add a little ingredient X, Paul wants you to add supplement Y, and for Caroline, cutting out Z is the key. But break it down and they are all saying the same things:

• Eat more fruit and vegetables

• Drink more water

• Eat more healthy fats

• Take some extra vitamin and mineral supplements

This is *Raw Living* in a nutshell. The basis of a raw food diet is raw fruit and vegetables, preferably organically and locally grown, and eaten seasonally. To that add liquids in the form of pure water and fresh juices; fats such as nuts, seeds, avocados, and olives; sprouted grains and pulses; and super foods like bee pollen and spirulina (a microalgae). You need to avoid meat, dairy, gluten, sugar, and all processed foods, but one of the joys of the raw food diet is that it is effective if you follow it at least 50 percent of the time. So you could have a raw breakfast, a cooked lunch, and a salad and something cooked for dinner, or eat raw all day and then have a cooked dinner. Chances are if you picked up this book, you are doing some of that already. See? Eating raw is easy, because it's intuitively what we want to do. You don't have to give up your favorite foods, but you will find over time that if you stick with it, your taste buds will change, and you will stop craving junk food and start craving super food!

I don't want to tell you what to do; there are enough experts around to do that. What I do want to do is to open the door to a whole new world of raw food cuisine. Raw foods are a revelation. After well over a decade of eating raw, I am more excited about this food than ever. I am still constantly discovering new ingredients or coming across new combinations. If I eat out at a raw friend's house, I am invariably delighted by the variety and individuality of their cuisine. Raw foods inspire us to fulfill our creative potential, both in the kitchen and out of it! Eating this way is a real pleasure: simple and easy to prepare, this food can be savored and enjoyed however busy your day, and fuel you with energy to cope with life's demands. When you eat foods that are fresh, locally, seasonally, and organically grown, you are tapping into the infinite life force of the earth, you are accessing divine energy, and it tastes good!

This collection of recipes consists of all the dishes that my family has particularly loved over the last few years. At the time I was creating them, I had three sons under the age of seven and little time or energy to spend slaving in the kitchen. I had to make sure the food was ready quickly, but I also had to make sure it was going to be eaten, and not left on the plate. So here they are, a unique collection of raw food recipes that will taste amazing, make you feel amazing, and still leave you with time to get out of the kitchen and on with your life.

I really loved writing this book. Going back to the information made me realize all over again how exciting raw foods are. It is such an easy concept to take on board, and its effects are nothing short of revolutionary. I have been traveling on this path for many years now, but it's human nature to take things for granted and forget how far we have come. These days I am in the blessed position where most of my friends and the people I surround myself with are raw fooders; it's not even something I think about anymore. Putting the information together for this book has helped me see it with fresh eyes.

I am passionate about the implications of the raw food diet for our society. When everyone starts to honestly take responsibility for their own health, to take their lives back into their own hands and empower themselves with the true facts about human potentiality and vitality, what kind of a world will we be creating then? When everyone wakes up feeling as super-charged and enthusiastic about life as the average raw fooder, what amazing realities will we be able to manifest? One of my most dearly held maxims is to "be the change you wish to see in the world." This is my main motivating force for eating a raw food diet, and why I feel it is so important. Eating raw provides us with one of the most integral tools for living a life of joy and abundance, for being a positive inspiration to those around us, and to counteracting all the negative and awful things that happen in the world day after day. I believe the best way to make the world a better place is to be a force for good in every way you can, at every moment possible; I believe complaining, fighting, and protesting just contributes more unhappiness to the overall global situation. After twenty years of thinking this way, I can see sure signs that humanity is beginning to see there is a bigger picture, and I am often overwhelmed by the massive shifts that could be made once this consensus becomes reality. Now we are at a time when this is truly possible, and by holding this book in your hands and accessing the information I have built up after years of study and experience, you have found a wonderful key for really making your life a shining example. How fantastic is that?

Conception and Pregnancy

*C*onception is the start of an amazing journey into parenthood, and the more you can do to prepare yourself and build a solid foundation, the easier it will be to spring into the chaos children bring into your lives. If you are at your optimum physically, it will enable you to conceive quickly, carry the baby successfully, give your child a great start in life, and build up your stores for the intensely depleting work of pregnancy and breastfeeding. For at least three months before starting to try for a baby, if circumstances allow, it is wise to examine your diet, your emotional well-being, and embark on a cleansing and detoxification program.

Like many young people, before I had children, I rarely got ill, had little stress in my life and few real responsibilities. I ate sensibly, but didn't give much thought to where I got my calcium or iron from. I didn't have a doctor. I don't remember even suffering from the occasional cold. So not only did the prospect of parenthood make me think seriously about how I was going to care for a child without following the conventional models, it made me reassess my own health provision. Carrying a baby puts untold stress on the body, and it doesn't stop at birth; breastfeeding demands huge amounts of physical resources too. Each time you have a child your body is left weakened and depleted, and unless you take a proactive approach to your health, each subsequent baby is likely to bring health complications as the stress of parenthood takes its toll.

On average, it takes a couple seven months to conceive. If you are fortunate enough to be in the position of actively trying for a baby, there are many simple dietary measures you can take to increase your fertility and ease the transition into motherhood. This isn't a time to be embarking on a radical healthy eating plan, but there are a few easy and gentle changes you can make. If you are too extreme, you will only yo-yo back to your old ways when you get pregnant, which puts stress on your body. If you go on a detoxing program when you are pregnant and breastfeeding, the baby can absorb the toxins that your body is getting rid of, through the placenta or in your milk, so it is wise to avoid cleansing at this time. Many women find it hard to keep up healthy eating habits when pregnant, particularly in the first trimester, so best to eat your greens now, before they make you throw up!

One of the most basic ways you can increase your fertility is to cut out alcohol, tobacco, and caffeine. In his book *Optimum Nutrition Before, During and After Pregnancy,* Patrick Holford cites research showing that drinking just one cup of coffee a day can halve your chances of conceiving, as can drinking alcohol daily, and that smoking damages the quality of your eggs and reduces the number capable of producing a baby. On the other hand, a diet high in antioxidants has been shown to aid fertility, especially in women over the age of thirty-five, so eating lots of raw fruit and vegetables is a must. Interestingly, both being underweight and overweight can lessen your chances of conceiving. In one study, nearly three-quarters of women with unexplained infertility conceived naturally once they stopped dieting and achieved their optimal weight. Conversely, if you are overweight, this can disturb your hormone balance and stop you ovulating. Losing just 10 percent of weight can dramatically stimulate ovulation.

The two essential minerals for fertility are selenium and zinc. Good sources of zinc are pumpkin seeds, chickpeas, cheese, and tahini. The best source of dietary selenium is Brazil nuts, which contain 839 micrograms (mcg) in 1 ounce of nuts (the RDA is 55 mcg!). Another good source is whole grains, such as wheat. However, due to intensive agriculture over the last century, and the extensive use of chemicals and pesticides on the land, our soil is generally depleted and doesn't contain the levels of minerals it used to, selenium being one of those minerals. On the vitamin front, B_6 is the one to watch out for. Vitamin B_6 is found in cauliflower, watercress, bananas, and broccoli. Also important is a daily dose of EFAs, which you can find in flaxseed and hemp oil. If you don't currently take any super foods, now is a really good time to start, for your baby's sake. Good ones for fertility are bee pollen (which is high in B$_6$ and zinc), and maca (*Lepidium Meyenii*), also known as nature's Viagra (see Super Foods on page 29).

Nausea in pregnancy is a result of the huge surge of hormones that pervade the body at this time. But in some primitive tribal cultures, morning sickness is unknown. I believe the degree to which you get sick is partially connected to how many toxins you have stored in your body, as well as emotional and lifestyle factors. Also affecting you is how much stress you are under during the pregnancy; stress creates toxicity in the system. You can help yourself by doing a liver cleanse before you try to conceive. Every morning for six weeks, first thing in the morning, take a tablespoon of olive oil mixed with a tablespoon of fresh lemon juice. It may not taste good to you and could well make you nauseous in itself, but it will help clear out congestion in the liver, and that should put you in good stead for what is to come. Wheatgrass is also an excellent liver cleanser. It is easy and cheap to grow your own, or you can buy ready-made trays from health food stores or online. Drinking 4 tablespoons of wheatgrass every morning is one of the best ways of detoxifying I have come across, because of its high chlorophyll content. Chlorophyll is exceptionally similar in composition to human blood, and oxygenates the cells. It is also fantastic for balancing blood sugar, and low blood sugar can be another cause of nausea.

It's vital to stay hydrated, especially if you are vomiting regularly. Many women find it next to impossible to drink pure water at the beginning. If you can't face it, try herbal teas, or some very diluted fruit concentrate; some women find carbonated water palatable when plain water is not. Ideally you should be aiming for at least 4 pints of liquid a day. Ginger and lemon are popular home remedies. Make some tea with grated ginger root, a slice of organic unwaxed lemon, and hot water, or if you have a juicer, add a piece of ginger (as much as you can stomach) and a slice of lemon and juice with apples and/or pears.

Once you've conceived, you're into a whole new unexplored territory foodwise. It's unfair, but at the time when eating healthily is probably more important than it has ever been in your life, it becomes very hard to control your desires for what you do and don't want to eat. I knew I was pregnant the second time because I developed a strong craving for Marmite on toast, neither foods that I usually eat; it was the exact same craving I had had with my first pregnancy. I'm sure it's no coincidence that Marmite contains beneficial vitamins and minerals for the developing fetus, and many women report it alleviates sickness. My body knew it wanted B vitamins, and knew where it had gotten them in the past, so it sent me in that direction. Many women find they want very bland and simple foods, without rich sauces, and however healthy you are, you are likely to find yourself craving junk foods—anything that's comforting and calming. It's important to strike a balance and look after yourself in all areas of your life as much as you can; this is likely to be your last chance to get leisure time for a few years! Don't be hard on yourself for wanting unhealthy foods and don't deny yourself what you want to make you happy, but balance the junk with some nutrient-dense foods that you still find palatable. The key to optimum health in this period is finding a few really nutritious foods that you love and making sure you get them down you as much as possible. You won't have much room in your stomach for big meals, but you need to keep your strength up, so keep the focus on juices and super foods. Eating raw is really not the priority: making sure you are sending your body all the love you can and feeding it vitamins and minerals any way you can is where your attention should go. Trying to be too controlling over your diet at this time is unhelpful and dangerous. If you haven't done the work on your health prior to conception, now is really not the time to be pushing yourself. Love yourself for exactly who you are, and revel in this unique and fascinating period in your life.

Breastfeeding

reastfeeding can be a wonderfully bonding experience for mother and baby, and it is truly amazing to watch your little one flourish on the miracle fluid your body makes. But it is really hard work! Whereas pregnancy demands only 300 extra calories a day from the body, breastfeeding demands about 500. And whereas pregnancy is a time to (hopefully) rest, nurture yourself, and bathe in the near universal good wishes of everyone around you, the commitment of breastfeeding is given little to no recognition in our society. You are literally giving of yourself usually for endless hours, day and night, while you are expected to competently carry on with all your other responsibilities too. No wonder most women give up before the first year is out. But there is no doubt that the longer you breastfeed, the better start your child has in life. In my experience, most children who are allowed to self-wean do so around thirty-six months old, although many go on longer.

So having just gone through the miracle of pregnancy and childbirth, when your body has really been put through its paces, it has to deal with this most demanding of tasks, maybe for several years. Most women find themselves ravenously hungry in the first few months after the birth. It is vital, for your health and that of the baby, that you take really good care of yourself. You might not get time to nurture yourself with long baths, uninterrupted time with your partner, or lazy Sundays, but you can eat well. In fact, it may be a welcome opportunity for you to eat as much as you like without having to worry about putting on weight!

Between the three boys, I breastfed continuously for nearly ten years, and was on a high raw diet throughout this time. I searched long and hard for the answers to good health that would help sustain me, and not leave me feeling exhausted and depleted. Raw foods have without a doubt been a major factor in allowing me to give my all to my children, and still have some energy left for myself. But they have their limits. Breastfeeding is so demanding on the body that you need to consume huge quantities of nutrients, and however carefully you eat, you're not going to be able to get enough from your food. Overeating is never good, puts a strain on your digestive system, and makes you tired and sluggish. In my opinion, the answers lie in super foods and juices, which when used correctly, give you sustained energy, without creating additional work for the body.

You need to ensure you're getting your protein, to help build baby's body up. Lots of sprouts are essential: lentil, chickpea, and mung bean are wonderful. Too many nuts and seeds can be mucus forming: if you overeat on them, particularly if they are not soaked first, you may find your child starts producing lovely thick green or yellow snot. The best ones to have are hemp, sesame, pumpkin, and sunflower, making sure they are soaked for at least a few hours. I always try to soak them overnight, and then leave them to sprout for a whole day if possible. Sesame is a powerhouse of nutrients: particularly needed for breastfeeding are calcium, iron, zinc, and the B vitamins, especially B_6. Zinc is really important. Good sources are pumpkin seeds, chickpeas, and tahini. B_6 can be found in cauliflower, watercress, bananas, and broccoli (one banana provides over 50 percent of the RDA), and don't forget the B_{12}—the only way to be 100 percent sure with that one is to take it in supplement form. As for calcium, breastfeeding women need a whopping 550 milligrams extra per day—look for it in green vegetables (particularly broccoli), seaweeds, sesame seeds, and maca.

You also need a good supply of fats to make lovely rich breast milk. Again, don't overdo the nuts and seeds, but do include raw oils such as olive and flax, as well as avocados and olives. Flax oil is always important in the diet, but never more so than at this stage: try to include 1–2 table-spoons a day. If you're not strictly raw you may want to include some molasses in your diet: rich in iron and calcium, it's very good mixed with tahini and spread on crackers and Essene (sprouted) bread. Nutritional yeast flakes are not a raw product either, but they are chock full of B vita-mins, and make a tasty addition to most dinners.

Some days, I used to feel very much like a cow: I did little but eat my greens and produce milk, going back and forth between baby and kitchen from morning to night, alternately grazing and being milked. My green juice is my wonder drink, my lifesaver, the tonic I absolutely could not do without. Never, since my discovery of raw foods, have I experienced such a profound shift in health as I did when I started on green juice every day. It took my diet onto a whole new level, partly because it is an excellent way of getting nutrients into the body, particularly the minerals that are so essential for breastfeeding. But equally beneficial are the deep cleansing and alkalizing properties of the juice that flood my system, keep me in balance, and help me to make better food choices throughout the day. I drink at least a pint a day, usually a combination of broccoli, fennel (which is good for milk production), celery, cucumber, and parsley (for iron). You can't beat some locally grown, in season greens such as spring greens, chard, or kale, or if you like your wild foods, dandelion and nettle are wonderful leaves to juice. I could not get enough broccoli: in one form or another, I had about 2 pounds a day. It's one of the most nutritious vegetables, and exceptionally high in calcium and the B vitamins.

Remember, you are effectively providing your baby with his first food, and if your diet is lacking, so is his. To ensure the good health of your baby, it is vital that you overcompensate, packing as much nutrition in you as possible, rather than risk leaving your child deficient. For this reason, super foods are really the only way to go. Super foods are natural plant foods that are incredibly dense nutritionally, and are much more easily assimilated by the body than artificially produced supplements. There is a huge variety to choose from these days, but the ones I recommend for breastfeeding are bee pollen and maca. Bee pollen has a delicious sweet taste, and gives you an instant energy hit, so you can have some whenever you start to flag. It's a complete food, containing all the vitamins and minerals essential to the body, but particularly noteworthy for moms because of its high levels of vitamin B_6 and zinc. Maca is great for balancing your hormones, and can help lift your mood and stave off hunger when you're sitting and feeding all day. It is also used for stamina and endurance, as well as being a complete protein and high in many vitamins and minerals, including calcium and zinc.

I also recommend drinking plenty of water. You may be shocked at first at the amounts you need to drink, but think of all those hours you sit feeding, and how much fluid is leaving your body in the form of breast milk. I personally used to drink 8 pints a day: two in the morning before breakfast, another two before lunch, another two in the afternoon, and two more before bed. It is very important to stay hydrated to ward off fatigue—I would say aim for at least 6 pints a day.

Breastfeeding is not discussed much because it's not something we will all do in our lives: even when you've discounted the male half of the population, many women don't have children, and many of those that do, choose not to, or can't, feed their babies themselves. But it is something that most of us experience, as newborns ourselves, and as such it is crucially important because it provides us with our physical foundation, as our little bodies build and grow. The nutrition that we receive in the womb and in the first few years at the breast can set us up for a lifetime of good health. It seems to me indisputable that all women who carry this great honor and responsibility should do the best they can to ensure the well-being of the next generation.

Children

*F*eeding children is a minefield, whether they're raw or not. When they're little, it's impossible to know what they want to eat, resulting in many wasted meals and frustrating feeding times. When they get older what they want isn't always what we would want for them! As raw foodists, it's made even harder by the lack of concrete information on suitable foods for children; there are so many differing opinions on what are the right foods for adults, and there has been virtually no research on how children's needs differ from ours. On the one hand, you might consider weaning your child on fruit, as it is easy to digest and easy to mash. But then you might worry about the amount of sugar in the diet, so consider vegetables instead. But raw vegetables are much harder to puree and not so tasty. Do you add in fats for sustenance, or are they too dense for children? What about sprouted grain crackers: do they make good finger foods, or are they too denatured for baby's sensitive palate? If you listened to all the "experts" you would end up feeding them nothing, but that is the last thing you want to do; you want a big, healthy well-fed baby to demonstrate to all the concerned relatives and health-care professionals how your offspring is thriving on your chosen diet and that you are a responsible parent.

I am sorry to say there is no simple answer. I wish I could say "give them this, this, and this," and all us moms could rest peacefully in our beds at night. The thing is children are their own people, with their own characteristics, and their own likes and dislikes. When Reuben was born, I had all these fixed ideas on how I was going to wean him, a carefully programmed, well-balanced diet, gently introducing him to a wide range of healthy raw foods. But he was having none of it, steadfastly refusing whatever I put in front of him unless it was cooked. What I learned is that children are our mirrors; whatever you eat while they are in the womb influences their taste buds, setting down their desires and cravings for their first few years. Reuben has a taste for cooked foods because I ate them when I was pregnant and breastfeeding; Ethan doesn't, but he has a very sweet tooth, as I was eating a lot of fruit when I was carrying and feeding him. As parents we are their role models; if they see one or the other of us eating cooked foods, you can be sure they will want some too. You can't set higher standards for your children than for yourself, it just doesn't work; if you have cooked foods in the house you are going to have to accept that they will be eating them too. So, like most things in life, it comes right back to where we are in ourselves. All we can do is to set the right example with what we eat, and sure as durian is durian, they will follow—eventually.

Don't spend your day in the kitchen trying to find something they relish, or you are creating issues around food. If you let them see that it is a big deal to you what they eat, they quickly catch on it is one of your "buttons" that they can press to wind you up—you are setting yourself up for power struggles and miserable mealtimes. On the other hand, don't starve them on a diet of grapes and cucumber; children need sustenance, they need reserves, because they're growing so fast. If there are one or two foods that they will eat, that seem to suit them, like bananas or avocados, don't worry, just let them get on with it—in a month or two they'll be on to something else. If they refuse everything you prepare, just make extras of what you have. Most children go through fussy stages where it seems like they're not eating anything; but no child will willingly starve themselves (they will also go through stages where they want to eat you out of house and home!). If you keep pandering to them and making them special dishes, they are going to keep demanding their own meals and creating a whole load of work for you. It's a hard balancing act, to make sure they're eating enough without making an issue out of it, but the trick really is to just let them see you enjoying your food, and they will want some too.

The secret of feeding healthy children is all the little extras that you can add in without them noticing. There are a number of things you can include in their diet that they will barely taste, but will really boost their nutritional levels. The two most important ones are water and flaxseed oil. I could write a whole chapter on the importance of getting enough of these, but suffice it to say that they will make a huge difference to your child's mood, energy, and ability to learn and concentrate. Few children drink enough water—every time mine are hungry, I tell them to have a cup of water first. So often we mistake the thirst signal for hunger. By the time they are five, you should be aiming for 2 pints a day, upping it to 4 by the time they are teenagers. Flax oil is the best vegan source of EFAs, the omega-6 and omega-3 oils. Most flax oils are processed in such a way to ensure that they are still raw. Children need at least a teaspoon a day, preferably a tablespoon. We can also find it in flaxseeds and hemp seeds, but it is much harder for the body to absorb. If you can't get them to take flax oil, you can always massage them with it; they will absorb it through the skin. We have lecithin with our flax oil: it contains phosphatidyl-choline, which helps with brain development, and it also aids in the emulsification of fats, enabling the body to absorb the EFAs better.

I am also a great believer in super foods. Our soil is so depleted now that even if we eat organic, the nutrient levels in foods are still much lower than they were just fifty years ago. Super foods are particularly invaluable for fussy children, acting as a safety net, so you know at least they've had something decent on those days when they don't want to eat. Bee pollen and Klamath Lake blue-green algae are both natural food sources that contain everything the body needs to sustain life. Children only need tiny amounts, so it needn't be costly: about $\frac{1}{4}$ teaspoon a day, or they will be too restless and unable to sleep.

Sea vegetables are the most mineral-rich foods that there are, and there's a wide variety to choose from. We have kelp powder (just $\frac{1}{4}$ teaspoon for the children), and sea salad (a blend of dulse, sea lettuce, and nori, made by Clearspring in Britain) or nori flakes on our lunch (alongside nutritional yeast flakes that aren't raw, but are a great source of B vitamins, and children seem to love the taste). For dinner, I often put arame (or "worms"!) in their salad. They love nori sheets (kids think it's great fun to eat paper; I remember I loved rice paper as a child), and a fun meal is to make a couple of tasty pâtés, put them on the table with some sprouts, and let them make their own nori rolls. Dulse and wakame make great seaweed chips if you rinse them (wakame needs soaking for 10 minutes) and put them in the dehydrator for about 6 hours, until crispy. While we're on the subject, tomato chips are another favorite in our family. We spread nut butter on them and sandwich two together.

For years, the boys' favorite was pasta—I cooked some rice or corn pasta and drowned it in raw pasta sauce (see recipe on page 150). They're happy because they're getting pasta for dinner; I'm happy because they're getting tomatoes, celery, carrots, avocado . . . Thankfully, I've weaned them off the cooked dinners now, but I've used this trick a lot in the past: they think they're getting a cooked dinner, when you know they're getting their quota of raw as well. I used to make a soup by cooking potatoes and onions, then adding some raw vegetables and almond butter and blending it all up. You can do this with rice, millet, lentils: cook as normal, and when done add vegetables, seaweed, and nut butter, whatever you can sneak past them. The other thing that works great if they want cooked food is bartering. Make a deal with them—if you eat a carrot, you can have a rice cake; if you eat a banana, you can have some yogurt. If they eat all their dinner, they can get a treat like a date or a sweet in the bath. This system is fantastic because it gets you out of arguments; they don't have to do what *you* want, but if they don't, they won't get what *they* want—it's simple, and it worked for me.

Most children will prefer fruit over vegetables, so you've really got to encourage them to eat those green leafies and steer them away from too much sugar. Try not to let them eat more sweet fruit than vegetables; if you let them fill up on the sweet stuff you are encouraging a sugar habit and mood swings that you definitely don't want in a two year old or a teenager! It's far better that they eat lightly cooked vegetables than none at all. Things like kale and broccoli are fantastic just steamed or stir-fried for a couple of minutes to soften them a little, and smothered in a creamy walnut dressing (see page 85). Avoid too much dried fruit because of problems with tooth decay. One good way to start the day is with a smoothie, and bigger children may take pride and pleasure in making their own. They can invent their own recipes—a banana, some seasonal fruits, their favorite nut butter or flax oil, and a cup of water to blend. Banana ice cream is another favorite of ours—peel bananas, break into chunks, freeze for 12 hours, and process, preferably in a high-power juicer, but a food processor or Vita-Mix will do. We had it for breakfast every day one summer—how fantastic is that, having ice cream for breakfast? When Ethan was going through one of his fussy stages, he had chocolate pudding (see page 178) with added flax oil and blue-green algae every day for lunch—and who can blame him, I had to stop myself from eating it all most days.

CHILDREN'S PARTIES

Christmas comes but once a year, birthdays however come once, twice, or maybe more, depending on the size of your family. At first, catering for a children's party can seem like every raw foodist's nightmare—the potential for conflicts over junk food is huge. In the early days I used to worry myself silly trying to prepare a feast that everyone would be happy with. Of course, you can't please all the people all the time, and despite my best efforts it never really worked. The main problem was that the more effort I put in, the more disappointed I was when people didn't appreciate, or even worse, didn't eat, my raw culinary creations. Or if I put "healthy" cooked food out, like rice cakes or vegan cookies, I would be annoyed when that was all my children wanted to eat, while their cousins, accustomed to junk food, wouldn't touch them at all.

In my experience, children aren't really that interested in food at parties. They want to run around making a noise and a mess, and have far too much energy to actually sit still for any length of time and eat anything. You usually need far less than you think you are going to. For instance, at Ethan's last party I was doing dips and only had two carrots to go round five children and three adults. Whereas previously I would have sent Chris out on an emergency trip to the shops, I just did what I had, and what do you know, there was still some leftovers at the end.

The basic plan is to keep it simple. Don't try too hard to impress people with your gourmet raw cuisine, because no one's going to be that bothered. As a general rule, don't put anything out that you don't mind your children eating a lot of. You can't argue about food in the middle of the party, and it would be mean to limit what they have—they need to feel that they can spoil themselves. So don't put out rice cakes unless you don't mind if that is all they end up eating. For older children, if they are absolutely adamant that they want chips, veggie sausages, or whatever they had at a friend's party, then just buy enough so there's only a little bit to go round and they can't overdose on them. But if you can get away with it, it's better to leave that stuff out altogether. You can bet that if you put out a big bowl of chips and a big bowl of carrot sticks, all the chips will get eaten and all the carrots will be left.

So just do the bare minimum. Dips are a basic that you can't go wrong with. Yellow, orange and red peppers, carrots, broccoli, and cucumber sticks for dipping are the most popular (celery always gets left). Do a couple of dips such as raw hummus, tomato ketchup, or tahini dip—one vegetable-based one and one nutty one for variety. Traffic light crackers are a winner (page 161). Arrange them on every child's plate before they sit down, to start them off. Replace fatty, salty, fried potato chips with tomato chips. If you're catering for adults as well, make a big green salad and you should be covered.

Personally, I would steer away from desserts. A gathering of children needs no encouragement in order to run around hyperactively. Too much sugar and there are bound to be tears. All you need is a fruit bowl so they can help themselves to grapes, apples, oranges, or bananas. If you're keen, you might want to make some sweets with nuts and dried fruit, or some dehydrated cookies. For Reuben's birthday one year, he was insistent that we make raw cupcakes. We made a cookie mix, some with oat groats and some with sprouted wheat (you could use the flapjack recipe on page 215 and just add a little extra water, 4 tablespoons would do, to make a cookie batter), and spooned it into little paper cases. When they were dehydrated the next day, we made a carob icing, and put a lexia raisin on the top for decoration. Jelly and ice cream might also be worth a try, although not for children used to dairy, sugar, and so on, who will probably find it too bland and reject your efforts. Make the ice cream from frozen bananas, and the jelly made from agar and juice or psyllium and pureed fruit. It's messy (make sure they sit at the table to eat it), but delicious.

Another idea that children love is to make little fruit kebabs (page 183). Buy a pack of cocktail sticks and assemble your chosen ingredients—you want a selection of dried and fresh fruit. Skewer them as close to eating time as possible, so they don't brown and become unappetizing. Get your children to help you put four or five items on the stick—the possibilities are endless, but try and get a mix of fresh and dried fruit on each. For some reason, children adore these little cocktail sticks, and have as much fun making them as they will eating them. If you don't mind the mess, you can make some carob sauce or cashew cream to dip them into.

But it's best to save your energies for the birthday cake, which really is your *pièce de résistance* and the one dish that everyone will remember. If you are having lots of children who aren't used to raw foods, a fruit tart is the most foolproof option. Make a crust with equal amounts of dates and almonds, and fill it with whatever fruit is in season. In the winter, you could slice apples and pears very thinly, and fill the crust with those. In the summer, a selection of berries makes a wonderful option—blackberries, raspberries, blueberries, and strawberries. Or you could try an exotic fruit combo such as mango and kiwi, two fruits that are always popular with children.

One more tip—always give tiny portions of cake. I find it very soul destroying to see all my wonderful food left over on party plates when all the children have taken a couple of mouthfuls and pushed it around the plate a bit. They can always come back for seconds, thirds, and even fourths! Psychologically, your children will feel a lot more indulged and spoiled if they have had three small portions of cake than one large one.

Finally, if you are inviting grannies and aunties to your party, who simply can't live without their cheese sandwiches, ask one special relative who enjoys catering if they could bring a big plate for everyone to share. Most people would prefer to do this than go hungry (or have to eat your rabbit food). If diplomacy is required, just explain that you will be doing lots of lovely food, but it's not the sort of thing that they usually eat, and would they like to bring a favorite dish (and maybe coffee or a few tea bags) in case they want something else.

Sample Menu

Traffic light crackers	Leafy green salad
Tomato chips	Birthday cake
Tahini dip	Ice cream and jelly
Tomato ketchup	Nuts and dried fruit sweets
Carrot, pepper, and cucumber sticks	Flapjacks
	Fruit kebabs and carob sauce

Husbands
(and Other Partners)

When I met my first husband, Chris, he was a vegetarian; over the course of five years he became 90 percent raw. When we were first together, he refused to have a salad for dinner because he claimed it wouldn't be substantial enough; I remember so clearly the day that came, when I said I was planning to do baby new potatoes with our dinner and he said, "I'd prefer to have something raw." So what happened along the way? Did I pester him, nag him, and badger him into going raw? Well, maybe a little! But everyone has to go on their own raw journey, and the beauty of raw foods is that they themselves are the best teachers.

Many women I speak to who come to raw foods after already having had a family, cite their husband's resistance to raw foods as one of the hardest obstacles to overcome. If you're uninformed, it's easy to dismiss it as another faddy diet, and see no reason to forsake all the favorite tastes to which you are accustomed. So women often try to carry on cooking for their men, but if you're anything like me, I find it impossible not to have a taste of something I'm making (just to check the flavors of course!). And if you're hungry and stressed and busy and tired, it's easy for that taste to turn into a few mouthfuls, or even dinner itself. So to make your life easier, if nothing else, you've got to show them that eating raw foods is something they want to do, as well as something they'll enjoy doing.

Men hate to be nagged. If they are going to eat raw, they must feel like it's their idea, that they are doing it because they genuinely want to. Not only will most men dig their heels in and rebel if they think that you're (literally) trying to shove something down their throats, no one's going to stick to it unless it's something they truly believe in. So leave some raw food books lying around for him to read—Juliano's *Uncook Book* if you think he'll be tempted by all the yummy pictures, or try *Conscious Eating* by Gabriel Cousens if he's more likely to be persuaded by scientific facts. Ask if he'll come to a lecture by an inspirational speaker such as David Wolfe or Shazzie. If he really won't listen to you, ring up one of the many raw food practitioners around who offer consultations and they can assuage his doubts.

Make sure he has plenty of choice, and enough to fill him up, or he is going to reach for the cooked treats and fall back into old habits. Make raw versions of his cooked favorites. If you are able, invest in a dehydrator; transitioning a family from cooked to raw without one is hard. I have my dehydrator on for about three days a week, for cookies, cakes, crackers, chips, burgers, loaves, and so on. These raw treats, made from sprouted grains such as oats, buckwheat, wheat, rye, and spelt, are a very satisfying alternative to conventional cakes and cookies. When grains are milled into flour and cooked, the gluten in them makes them hard to digest, and plays havoc with blood sugar levels; sprouting releases enzymes that turn the starches into more easily digestible sugars, as well as increasing the nutritional content.

So hopefully by now, he's seen the sense in it, even if he still might not be keen to try it himself. In my experience, the best way to proceed is by compromise. For dinner every day, make one cooked dish and one raw dish. Give yourself a large portion of raw (and a small portion of cooked if you want), and give him his usual cooked portion, with a small raw side dish. Make something really tasty, but only give him a little bit—leave him wanting more! Gradually, over the weeks and months, up the raw quotient, until one day you'll be able to leave out the cooked altogether.

Chris didn't need me to go on at him about the benefits of raw foods, because he started to feel them for himself. We are always talking about cooked foods being addictive—they are, for sure, the hardest addiction to fight. Recent research from the University of Wisconsin shows that junk food alters brain biochemistry with effects similar to drugs such as morphine, nicotine, or heroine! But you get hooked on raw foods too. When you have those days when you feel as light as a feather, your energy is soaring, and even when things go wrong you just know that it must have happened for a good reason; that feeling is addictive. We went to a party a few years back, and there was a lot of raw food, but also lots of vegan cake and ice cream. Chris ate loads of cake, but I didn't care—I knew he'd have a cooked food hangover the next day, and that he'd know for himself that he didn't want a wife who baked! All you can do is trust that if you guide your husband gently on to the path, if he's got any sense at all, he'll be leaping along the way in no time, and maybe even overtake you!

And if you're a male raw fooder reading this book, and you're saying, "What about me?" I say, "Wow, isn't your lady lucky?" There's a lot of raw women around who find it hard to find a man who is as into looking after their bodies as they are. If you're already in a relationship, your partner is very fortunate to be with such a switched-on guy. And if you're single, you've got your pick of the raw goddesses to choose from.

Aphrodisiacs

*T*he public image of the raw food diet is changing. A few years ago when I told people I ate a raw diet, the most common question would be "What do you eat?" And when I told people the sort of things we had for dinner—burgers, Thai, pasta, sushi, not to mention the cakes, puddings, and ice cream—they would be astounded. The common belief was that you had to live on apples and lettuce and not a lot else. One woman actually came to a workshop to find out more and said, "Oh I thought it was going to be ten ways to peel a banana." But raw foods' time has come, and thanks to the dozens of high-quality raw recipe books and Internet sites around now, people are seeing how interesting and varied a raw diet can be.

Look at anyone who has followed a raw food diet consistently for a few years or more, has done their share of detoxing, purged a few inner demons, sloughed away some dead cells, and is on the road to optimum health. See how they glow with an inner radiance and vitality no amount of expensive beauty products can achieve. See the way they are so comfortable in their bodies, with a natural confidence that is incredibly attractive. See how they fully inhabit themselves, how they have a brighter, a more whole aura that is very affirming and healing to be around. Have a look at some of the raw movies on YouTube, the online video channel, and you'll see what I mean.

So how do you get some of that magnetic charisma for yourself? Well first of all, it has to be said that it does take years of dedication. Going raw for a short while isn't hard at all, but if you want to reap the full benefits, keep at it year after year and you'll be amazed as the old layers of yourself peel away, revealing the nakedly raw, gloriously true you! It's a very liberating process. And it involves far more than just dietary changes, but encompasses a whole outlook on life—regular exercise, holistic therapies, helpful cleansing techniques, and most importantly a shift in consciousness. Eating the raw way, nature's way, is one of affirmation, abundance, joy, and vitality, and it's only going to work if you feed your mind the same high-quality foods as your body, focus relentlessly on the positive, and try at all times to make the world a better place for you and everyone around you, thereby healing our beautiful planet. Honestly, there is nothing more sexy than an inner knowing that you are following your path, living true to your heart, and fulfilling your mission to create a more peaceful, loving world. The closer to nature you are, the more tuned into your body and the planet, the more you exude a wild, liberated, fecund energy that is very intriguing to people and will draw them to you.

So you've been listening to your body and energizing your life, and you've attracted a delicious mate, what are you going to feed them? Making food together is always a good start. Raw food preparation is very sensual. Roll up your sleeves and get stuck in there. Use your hands to toss the salad; use your fingers to scrape the jug; really massage that kale, knead that raw cookie dough, and whip that cashew cream. Lots of licking fingers and feeding each other tastes off spoons works wonders to get the libido going.

• Maca is the number-one aphrodisiacal food. With a not unpleasant, malty kind of taste, it is easy to add to most kinds of sweet dishes. Try some in your oatmeal or your yogurt, sprinkle it on your cereal, add it to smoothies, or make a spread with it and plaster it over your sprouted bread and dehydrated crackers. A simple summer recipe is to blend up 1 tablespoon of maca with a couple handfuls of strawberries, a banana, and a splash of natural sweetener such as agave nectar. It is brilliant for extra energy and stamina—it provides a calm, centered, and long-lasting boost. As a powerful hormone balancer, it restores the body's natural libido—it is often called nature's Viagra.

• Everyone loves chocolate but wait until you try it in its raw naked form —you will be blown away. It contains natural chemical compounds that boost serotonin levels and produce a real natural high. And of course, it helps the body to produce feel-good hormones that are a great natural aphrodisiac. Try one of the sublime raw chocolate bars that are starting to appear in whole food stores, and are sugar-free, wheat-free, and dairy-free. Or even better, track down some cacao nibs and make your own (page 220). Making chocolate is like therapy—the aromas and the textures are incredibly sensual and very healing. Throw some maca in the mix and wow! Guaranteed fun.

• Maybe you prefer savory foods over sweets? The raw fooders favorite snack food is nori rolls. Get some raw nori sheets (not the toasted ones) and cram with creamy dips like hemp seed hummus (page 63), almond mayonnaise, or cacaomole (guacamole with extra chocolate—really, it works). Sprinkle in some fresh wild herbs and locally sourced greens like arugula and spinach, layer in some alfalfa sprouts and roll. Share with your partner, one end each. Packed with minerals, this kind of food is very strengthening, and somehow there's something very sexy about bits of avocado spilling out of your mouth and dribbling down your chin. Nori rolls can't be eaten politely—you have to abandon yourself to them and that's all part of the fun.

• One of the simplest and most effective aphrodisiacs is a good old-fashioned brew. Some herbs have been used for centuries for their nurturing and reviving properties. A cup of tea like this after your dinner is sure to have you heading straight for the bedroom—in fact, you might not even make it that far. . . . Try one of the blended brands on the market, or look out for herbs such as yohimbe, damiana, or bala.

Now excuse me, after all that I'm off to find myself a handsome raw man who has so much energy and stamina he can keep going all night and still be up in the morning to feed me exotic fruit and freshly made juice—or even some more chocolate . . .

Super Foods

I love super foods. I eat them every day, and have done so for nearly two decades. I don't know how I could survive without them—sure, I would still be alive, but I think I can state categorically that I would not be as happy and energetic without them, and I certainly wouldn't be leading such a joyful and abundant life. They provide me with that edge, that get-up-and-go that helps me deal with the demands of motherhood and still have energy for myself. As a breastfeeding mother, I could be sure my high nutritional requirements were being met. And when my children are fussy and push away the green vegetables on their plates, I can rest assured they will get their greens one way or another!

Although most people have heard of super foods, there is some confusion over what the term actually means. I would classify them as natural plant foods that are exceptionally high in nutrition and thereby provide the body with increased energy. Broccoli and blueberries are not super foods. They may be very healthy food choices, but they don't have the supercharged density and vitality of true super foods. True super foods really can transform you into a super being. Because all the vitamins, minerals, amino acids, enzymes, fatty acids, and more are so packed in, a little goes a long way. A lot of energy is saved on the digestion process, and if taken correctly and the body is functioning well, they are easily absorbed and assimilated, thus providing an instant boost. Super foods are generally superior to supplements because they are literally a whole food. Anything that has been synthesized in a laboratory or chemically isolated is not going to send the body as strong and clear a message as a natural plant food that has simply been dried or powdered. This is one reason why super foods are gaining popularity so quickly: you definitely notice when you take them, and you can really feel the difference.

Many super foods grow in poor, isolated, but unspoilt regions such as in Peru and Tibet. They are well-known in their native countries and have been eaten for centuries by the indigenous populations, but no one has properly looked into their nutritional benefits and properties before. With the demand for healthy food options increasing in the West, and the whole foods market being one of the biggest retail growth sectors, much research is now being done in the search for innovative new products, and many amazing new foods are being discovered and brought to us. So you may read on and think, "But I've never heard of any of these foods!" That's because many of them have only been easily available here for a year or two, sometimes even less. But word is spreading fast about their amazing health benefits and you can bet you'll soon be seeing goji berries next to the Mars bars on supermarket checkouts.

The most well-known super foods currently are algae (spirulina, Klamath Lake blue-green algae, and chlorella), bee pollen, and aloe vera. Wheatgrass is also widely recognized for its health benefits, but people are less likely to have it regularly because ideally it is consumed freshly juiced. Some of the newer ones that have been around a couple of years now are cacao, maca, and goji berries. And then we have the really new kids on the block like suma, camu camu, purple corn, noni juice, crystal manna, and more. . . . There are a lot of super-food blends on the market too, in which anything from 10–100 high-potency foods are powdered together. Basically, I would say that old adage is true: "you get what you pay for." If one brand is less expensive than another, it probably has cheaper ingredients and fillers in it. Generally, all these blends are quite costly and not optimum because they have been put through a greater degree of processing to reach you. Many of them contain a large number of different ingredients, and it can be overwhelming for the body to be bombarded with complicated messages in this way. No super food is a bad super food, and they can all be helpful, but some more than others!

It is very hard to compare the different qualities of the super foods that we use; it's a bit like trying to compare a carrot with a parsnip or a cabbage. They each have their own distinctive individual character, so people often have a particular aversion to one but get on really well with another. The correct dosage is also hard to predict. It is always best to start off with a little, say half a teaspoon, at least for the first couple of days. You may notice a reaction right away and like it—in which case up the dose! If you don't notice anything, you probably need more, so again, gradually up the dose until you start feeling the effects. If you notice a detox reaction such as an old complaint flaring up, pimples, or tummy troubles, this is just the body rebalancing, so stick with a minimum maintenance dose and after a few days you should have shifted some stuff and be feeling much better.

- Algae are the oldest life-form on earth—"primordial food." When we eat algae we connect with that really ancient energy. It is a very deep healing, but gentle food, and a good one to start with. There are three classes of algae widely available: chlorella, spirulina, and Klamath Lake blue-green algae. Spirulina is the best source of protein, but Klamath Lake is on the whole nutritionally superior. The Klamath Lake is in Oregon, it is a nutrient trap, and the algae that grow in it are some of the finest foods available to us. They are nutritionally complete, which means they contain absolutely every known nutrient the body needs. Not only that, they are in the ideal ratios for bioavailability. If you had to sit down and design the perfect food, blue-green algae would be hard to beat.

- Bee pollen is also a complete food. If you were stranded on a desert island with nothing but bee pollen and water, theoretically you would have everything you needed (although I don't think anyone's ever tested it out!). Bee pollen is a bit of a misnomer, because although it is collected by bees on their legs, it actually comes from flowers. It's a great one for kids because it has a naturally sweet taste, like honey; my boys have it on their cereal every morning. It is very energizing, good for those days when you have a dozen errands to run before school pick-up, and you need to be buzzing around all day.

- Aloe vera comes from a cactus plant and is usually drunk like a juice. The quality of aloe vera on the market is quite variable—if it tastes like water it probably is. Aloe is a truly amazing plant: as well as having a strong nutritional profile, it has antiviral and antimicrobial properties, and is a natural painkiller. Much research is being conducted in the United Kingdom on aloe at the moment, due to its widely reported benefits with both skin conditions like eczema and psoriasis, and gut problems such as irritable bowel syndrome (IBS) and colitis. Because of its immune-boosting properties, it is taken by many people suffering from immune disorders from asthma to lupus and cancer. And if all that wasn't enough, it is also popular with those suffering with joint problems, particularly athletes and the elderly.

• Wheatgrass is tops for detoxifying and cleansing as it is exceptionally high in chlorophyll. Chlorophyll has a very similar composition to human blood: you could call it plant blood, and as such, it is very healing. It is best consumed freshly juiced, for which you need a good-quality juicer, or you can find it at many juice bars; the powdered versions don't really compare. It is one of the most potent foods you will ever find, very good at balancing blood sugar and used to treat serious diseases such as cancer and diabetes.

• Cacao is known as the food of the gods. Native to South America, it is the bean that cocoa solids are made from, so it is literally raw chocolate. It is one of the highest dietary sources of magnesium and sulfur, as well as containing an off-the-chart level of antioxidants. It is full of natural chemicals that boost the mood and elevate energy levels, so providing an unbeatable natural high. Plus (unlike wheatgrass) it tastes wonderful—a luxurious sweet treat you can pig out on, and then feel heavenly afterwards, surely the answer to every woman's dreams . . .

• Maca is a Peruvian root vegetable that is most commonly found in powdered form. It is a great source of protein and minerals such as calcium and iron. It is a hormone balancer, so it is great for premenstrual syndrome (PMS), acts as a natural form of hormone replacement therapy (HRT), and is used to treat osteoporosis. It is also the number-one super food for pregnant and breastfeeding mothers, to help boost energy and stamina. It's even a natural aphrodisiac so it's good for making babies too.

• Goji berries are perhaps the most accessible super food. They come from one of the purest places on earth, the Himalayas, and are the most nutrient-dense fruit on the planet. They come to us dried, like raisins, but they taste far better. They contain all the essential amino acids, so they're a great source of protein, as well as being one of the highest natural sources of beta-carotene and vitamin C. Children love them: we eat them all day long, in our cereal for breakfast, in trail mixes, in smoothies, in puddings, cakes, salads, or just as they are. In China they say the only side effect to eating too many gojis is laughing too much.

So, I hope this introduction to the irresistible world of super foods has whetted your appetite. There are so many to try, they couldn't be easier to incorporate into your existing diet, and they are absolutely, undeniably beneficial—I truly believe that there's something wonderful there for everyone to discover.

Supporting Techniques

*E*ating raw is by no means the be all and end all of good health. There are plenty of unhealthy raw fooders around to prove that point! A lot of people try and go "100 percent raw" and then after a year or two, they say it can't be done, because it didn't work for them. It's very common for people to go raw and for the first few months feel fantastic, better than they have in years. But if eating raw is not part of a whole lifestyle package, it's impossible to sustain at that level. That's why I believe it's important at the beginning to keep it in balance: see it as a long-term goal, maybe five or ten years. There are no doubt a few exceptions around, but generally no one manages to go 100 percent raw and then stay there! Sometimes problems surface quite quickly; other times it can take years for long-suppressed issues to arise.

The key factor in all this is your state of mind. Where is your consciousness at? Raw foods are so full of vitality, they make one feel much more alive, and more present in the moment. We open up to that natural state of joy, love, and abundance that is our birthright. But it is very hard in our culture to sustain that vibration. Raw foods have a very high vibrational level; super foods even higher. So when we eat like this, we are opening ourselves up to these levels. And every single one of us has issues that need working on, fears and self-doubts that block our energy. So if we are not actively engaged in personal development, if "being the change that we want to see in the world" is not our motivating factor, then raw foods are not going to work for us. We are going to need to eat foods of a lower vibration to help us feel grounded and in our bodies and not spaced out.

For most people who are drawn to raw foods, creating a better world is part of their worldview. But often it is just one thread in a busy and complex life. Holding together the day-to-day responsibilities of a career, home, and family are the preoccupying concerns for most of us; the food we eat needs to support us in that, give us energy to fulfill our potential and to make the most out of life. Hence I emphasize the importance of "being where you're at" with raw foods, and not pushing it to extremes, because that is not holistic. If you're stressing over whether to eat some food that maybe isn't an optimum health choice, I say eat it; it's far better to enjoy the food rather than create stress in your life, or even worse, repress and deny your instincts. Our thoughts have the power to shape our lives; be mindful of yours.

Everyone knows that exercise is equally vital to a healthy lifestyle. If you're too busy to fit any into your daily routine, there is something out of balance in your life. If you're pressed for time, rebounding is great; just 5 minutes can tone the whole body and help stimulate the lymphatic system. Rebounding is basically just bouncing on a mini trampoline. It's fun to do to music, or even while you're watching TV. It places no strain on the joints, boosts circulation, and improves muscle tone. I often stop for rebounding sessions between writing chapters to loosen things up and keep the brain fresh. Yoga is very popular among raw food devotees: the two have a naturally symbiotic relationship. Both are about tuning into one's body, achieving a union between the higher and lower self. Many yoga students turn to raw food because they find it helps them get more flexible, and go further into their meditation; many raw fooders discover yoga as an ideal way to keep vibrant and attuned. Whatever exercise suits you best, swimming, walking, or cycling to work every day, if you consider it as vital a part of your daily routine as taking a shower and brushing your teeth, your body will love you for it.

Water is the most vital requirement for human life. The purer the water we drink, the better we can assimilate nutrients and flush out toxins. The quality of the water you drink is more important than any of the food you put into your body. You can eat the healthiest foods on the planet, but if you are not drinking enough water, your body will not be able to absorb and utilize the nutrients from the food. We use water that has been put through a unique process of reverse osmosis filtration and deionization (patented by Aquathin). Reverse osmosis is a process developed by NASA that squeezes water through a semipermeable membrane under pressure, rejecting impurities such as heavy metals, viruses, and hormones. The membrane is so fine, only hydrogen and oxygen molecules can pass through. Next, the water goes through a deionization process, which removes more impurities, and finally it passes through a granular activated carbon filter, which has great abilities to absorb many of the organic contaminants found in water.

I am a great believer in colonics and enemas. Some people dismiss them as unnatural, but I feel there is so much about our modern lifestyles that is unnatural that these deep-cleansing techniques are vital for keeping our bodies in balance. To me, cleaning my colon is as basic as cleaning my outer body: I couldn't go for more than a few days without a bath or a shower before I started feeling dirty, and if I go too long without colon cleansing I feel a similar unclean feeling. We accumulate so much waste matter in our guts; one colonic hydrotherapist told me that the most common substance found is mother's milk. Another told me you could have a colonic every day for a year before you stopped pulling stuff out; we produce so much waste matter continually. We are literally carrying around a lifetime's debris inside us. I recommend doing enemas at least once or twice a month, and having a colonic at least once or twice a year. I find the most beneficial times for cleansing are around the equinoxes and solstice, so choose to have them then if you can. Colonics are performed by registered practitioners in hygienic surroundings. They are more thorough than enemas, and clean higher up the colon. Enemas can be self-administered in your own home. They may feel strange at first, but with a bit of practice they become easy, quick, and not at all uncomfortable. Enema bags can easily be purchased online. I like to do two in a row; the first with just plain water and some essential oils such as lavender, eucalyptus, or peppermint, for cleansing; then I do a second containing nutritional substances that can be absorbed directly through the colon walls. I usually put in a probiotic to help build healthy gut bacteria, and MSM (naturally occurring sulfur crystals), which assists with absorption and increases overall body flexibility. Then I add a super food such as aloe vera, spirulina, barleygrass, or noni juice, as well as some hemp or flax oil to get an extra dose of EFAs. Each enema takes about 20 minutes in total (I have an enema information video on YouTube if you want more information). It doesn't matter how healthily we eat, our bodies are continually stressed by pollutants in the environment and in our lifestyles, and it seems to me that enemas are one of the simplest and most effective ways of dealing with the toll twenty-first-century living takes on our bodies. They are excellent ways of building digestive fire too, as retaining the water strengthens the muscles in the colon walls and teaches the gut to work more efficiently. So many people in our culture suffer from problems like IBS and colitis, which could often be easily remedied by a colon-cleansing program. Our guts have been weakened by decades of wrong eating and a buildup of debris and waste matter, no wonder they can't cope any more with the demands put on them. It doesn't matter how healthily you are eating if the cell walls in the gut are so clogged up you are not absorbing any nutrients!

As we become more conscious about the foods we put in our bodies, we begin to wonder about all the other things our bodies come into contact with too. There are an incredible number of pollutants in the environment, many of which can be reduced very simply. Here's just a few of the ways you can "detox your world" (as a good friend of mine once said):

• Use more natural products on your hair and skin, not ones full of unpro-nounceable chemicals. There are many excellent animal-free and organic products around. Look for ingredients like aloe vera, lavender or rose oil, hemp, MSM, and cacao butter, and check that what you are buying contains significant quantities of these special plant products, not just a token splash.

• Buy clothes and linen made with natural fibers, organic cotton or hemp, if possible. The chemicals used in growing cotton are some of the biggest pollutants on the planet, and cause massive health problems for the growers and pickers. Organic is more expensive, but it is becoming more accessible, and feels wonderful on the skin. Hemp is one of the most durable fabrics around and is amazingly soft to wear. It is good for the soil, uses little water, and needs no pesticides. Again, nowadays there is a growing range of hemp clothes made by young ethical designers— you can even buy hemp lingerie.

• Be aware of electromagnetic pollution, try to minimize the use of electri-cal equipment, and use protection devices wherever possible. I believe that the invisible pollution we are all bombarded with in the twenty-first century is one of the biggest potential health hazards we face. No one yet knows the consequences of the extensive use of computers, mobile phones, cordless phones, satellite navigation systems, and so on. Undoubtedly all these things make our lives much easier and more pleasurable, but they also potentially have hidden side effects. Leading a holistic lifestyle involves keeping all these devices in balance and using protective materials like crystals, or ones that have been specifically devised to protect against electromagnetic pollution like tachyon devices and plasmonic plates. Although your inner cynic might not be convinced there is enough evidence that these things actually work, I feel it is better to be overcautious and invest in whichever gadgets you are drawn to.

- Avoid unnecessary antibiotics, vaccinations, and other pharmaceutical products, and seek out natural therapies like homeopathy, flower essences, and acupuncture. Please don't get me started on the horrors of the pharmaceutical industry. If you want more information, a good place to start is www.naturalnews.com, an independent website that contains a real wealth of information on natural health, nutrition, and more. Many of the illnesses that we take medication for can be just as easily corrected with natural remedies. When we get ill, it is our body's way of clearing stuff out, and telling us to slow down and rest a bit. Allopathic medicine merely suppresses symptoms and does not help the body detoxify fully. Indeed, conventional medicine tends to weaken the immune system because it does not allow the body to do the work itself, but does the job of fighting disease for it. Alternative therapies, on the other hand, support the body in releasing toxins and make it stronger and healthier in the long term. And don't wait until you are ill to have a treatment; invest in your health continually. It is much more enjoyable having a preventative massage or Reiki session than having to drag yourself off somewhere for a consultation when you are feeling run-down and terrible.

- Invest in air ionizers and purifiers, and keep windows open as much as possible to ensure circulation of fresh air. If you have windows closed all the time, this leads to a buildup of carbon dioxide; open windows allow oxygen to circulate, making you feel more energized and alert. In the winter, try and avoid having the central heating on unnecessarily; it is very dehydrating and contributes to creating a sluggish system. It's far better to make your internal fire work a bit by feeling the cold, than allowing it to get lazy by adjusting the temperature artificially.

There are many easy-to-practice home remedies to assist the body in releasing toxins. Once you've been on a high raw diet for a few months, your body is going to start releasing a lot of old "stuff." People usually find it is around the three-month mark that things start to get moving for them. Often, people can take up a healthy habit for three months, but when it gets to the point where stuff is starting to shift for them, if they don't feel supported in making the appropriate changes in their lives, they fall back into old patterns. That is why detoxification techniques are so important, to enable the whole body to move forward, rather than just focusing on the one area like diet and then the rest of the body struggles to keep up.

There are lots of ways to ensure you have beautiful, radiant, naturally healthy skin. Your skin will love you if you have regular steams or saunas, which help open the pores and release toxins. Steam rooms are better because they use wet heat; saunas use dry heat, which is more dehydrating. Whichever you take, make sure to drink plenty of water during the session. Skin brushing helps to stimulate the lymphatic system, remove dead skin cells, and also leaves your skin looking great. You can buy a dry bristle brush from a health food store or drugstore; simply brush toward the heart, with long, hard strokes, before showering. Cold baths and showers are amazing; I have been taking cold showers for around fifteen years, and cold baths for around five years. I never notice the cold now, and I am sure this is largely because this daily boost to my circulation means I have built up a strong inner fire. The best way to shower is to run the shower cold first for as long as you can stand it; then have a usual hot shower and wash; then do alternate cold/hot/cold/hot/cold to end, always finishing with the cold. Cold baths are even more stimulating: after you've had your usual soak in a hot tub, drain the water out and remain in the bath. Then refill the bath with cold water, and stay in as long as you can, submerging your head and body completely if possible. Not only does this really get your system working full power, it's great for the mind too, as you're going beyond the usual limitations you set for yourself and breaking down barriers to what you believe is possible. Your head tells you, "I can't do this, it's too cold!", but if you push it and don't listen to that voice, you realize that you can do it, and really it isn't that bad after all. So often in life it's our belief that we can't do something that stops us achieving it, and techniques like this help us to create a positive attitude and inner mastery of situations.

Bathing in Epsom salts is an excellent way to remove toxins from the body. The salts draw acidic wastes out through the pores of the skin, and they also have a high magnesium content, a mineral many of us are lacking in. You need to put about 2 cups (500 g) of Epsom salts in a bath, and they are easily found in drugstores.

Another simple home remedy for drawing out toxicity is the use of castor oil packing: castor oil has antimicrobial and antibacterial properties and due to its full-spectrum-light content is excellent at pulling rubbish out of the body. Again, castor oil is cheap and easy to find in most drugstores. Simply soak an old flannel or muslin cloth or some special packing fabric in the oil, and place on the area where you want to achieve results. Liver packing is very beneficial, also packing on your lungs when you have a chest infection can be very helpful. Place a hot water bottle on top of the pack so the heat can help with the process. Settle down with a book or in front of a film for a couple of hours, or wear overnight while you sleep. Castor oil stains, so wear old clothes and sheets, or use plastic bags to cover the packing fabric and avoid it getting in contact with other materials. I love castor oil packing; it is wonderfully nourishing, nurturing, and soothing.

Finally, I highly recommend the work of Barbara Wren and the College of Natural Nutrition, which she founded. Barbara was a nurse who suffered from anorexia nervosa when she was younger and ME (myalgic encephalopathy or chronic fatigue syndrome) later in life. She had four children, and took her own journey to find optimum health. Her philosophy incorporates a high raw diet, as well as naturopathic techniques like castor oil packing and enemas, and observing the cycles of the moon and the sun. I love her methods particularly because they are generally so low-cost and easy to do, but have such far-reaching effects on our health.

The Journey

*P*eople are attracted to raw foods for many different reasons. Most commonly, people just want more energy; some want to lose weight, others to correct a medical condition like IBS or clear up a skin condition. Some have a serious health challenge such as cancer, others are perfectly healthy and want to stay that way. But whatever your motivation, raw foods are in themselves a journey, and I believe, a very spiritual journey. Eating raw opens you up to your true self; it helps you to look honestly at your life and the people in it. It's a common complaint among raw fooders that they find it hard to tell a lie! Being raw is a process of stripping away the layers of cooked food addiction; the fears, doubts, and insecurities we have about ourselves are laid bare, and at first we can feel quite exposed. But the more we get accustomed to being in our raw, naked state, and shed those false skins of protection, the more liberated we feel. This kind of liberation is like medicine; it might not always taste good, but it sure makes you feel better!

When I look at my own personal growth through raw foods it astounds me. I never worry about my weight now, whereas that was a major preoccupation throughout my teenage years. I always eat as much as I want and I never feel overweight. I have limitless supplies of energy, and need on average only 6 hours of sleep a night. I don't get tired despite my 110 m.p.h. lifestyle—three children, a thriving business, and a busy social life. Because I feed myself only the highest quality plant foods this amazing planet has to offer, I love my body and it rarely lets me down. My thoughts always tend toward the positive; because my food is so full of life energy, so am I. Sure, I have challenges and crises in my life, that's all part of being human, but I now have the confidence to know I will get through them, and a faith in the universe that leads me to understand everything happens for a reason, and there is always a valuable lesson to be learned in every situation. I am relentlessly happy and upbeat, almost to the point of being annoying, and feel gratitude in my heart for my life and all the amazing people in it. I am so at peace with myself, I feel the joy bubbling over on a daily basis. And so I attract fewer and fewer people into my life who judge me, disrespect me, or misunderstand me. Instead I draw in people who appreciate me and recognize my contribution to humanity. The more I surround myself with these amazing people, the happier I get, and the more beautiful beings I pull in!

This can work for you because you are eating foods that have a pure and harmonious energy, so you too start to create more of these energies in your life. When you are living in the present, in the moment, you are tuned in to yourself and your life's higher purpose and miracles start to manifest daily. It can just be little things like making it to the car one minute before the traffic officer comes round the corner, or a friend turning up with just the book or CD or raw cookies that you had been thinking about. But it can also be major life changes like finding a new partner, taking a new career path, or moving house. It's a fundamental universal law at work: the more bliss you find in your food, the more bliss you create in yourself, the more bliss you attract into your life.

Raw foods were an integral part of the journey to get me to this space. And no matter what the reality of your initial motivation for going raw, this is where it will lead you if you follow the path: to a place of love, joy, abundance, and vitality. It's what I call "raw magic." But that's a whole other story . . .

Sample Menus

*H*ere are some ideas to get you started and give you a good idea of what is possible on the raw diet. If you follow these menus for two weeks, you'll be so full of good food you won't be going hungry, but you're also likely to have more energy than ever and feel fantastic. Most people find that after a few months, weeks, or even days of eating good-quality raw food meals their appetites start to diminish and they are happier with simpler dishes and smaller meals, but if you're seeking to banish the cooked food cravings and keep fully raw, following these menus will be really helpful guidelines for you.

DAY ONE

Breakfast—cereal★

Mid-morning—1 chocolate brownie★

Lunch—Reuben's guacamole★, carrot sticks,
fresh arugula in red pepper dressing★

Mid-afternoon—seasonal fruit

Dinner—spicy almond burgers★ with red pepper ketchup★
and fennel and leek salad★

DAY TWO

Breakfast—breakfast pudding★

Mid-morning—2 sand crackers★

Lunch—beetroot soup★

Mid-afternoon—zucchini chips★ and Zachary's dip★

Dinner—red cabbage and apple salad★ and mashed parsnips★

★ Denotes that there is a recipe in the book for this dish.

DAY THREE

Breakfast—fresh juice made with $\frac{1}{2}$ cucumber,
2 sticks celery, and $\frac{1}{2}$ lemon

Mid-morning—dulse chips★ and cilantro chutney★

Lunch—rye bread★, alfalfa sprouts, and cashew cream cheese★

Mid-afternoon—seasonal fruit

Dinner—"chicken" salad★

DAY FOUR

Breakfast—"can't beta it"★

Mid-morning—raw chocolate★

Lunch—seasonal green salad leaves and sunflower sprouts
in creamy cucumber dressing★

Mid-afternoon—2 oatcakes★ and pumpkin seed butter

Dinner—chili★

DAY FIVE

Breakfast—cereal★

Mid-morning—seasonal fruit

Lunch—walnut pâté★ and carrot and pepper sticks

Mid-afternoon—fresh juice made with $\frac{1}{2}$ cucumber,
2 celery sticks, 1 apple

Dinner—dahl★

DAY SIX

Breakfast—miso bread★ and tahini

Mid-morning—maca balls★

Lunch—nori rolls stuffed with parsley dip★,
cucumber sticks, and alfalfa sprouts

Mid-afternoon—seasonal fruit

Dinner—lentil and sage sausages★ and carrot ketchup★
and fresh corn salad and avocado dressed in tapenade★

DAY SEVEN

Breakfast—gorgeous Goji pudding★

Mid-morning—2 lovely biscuits★

Lunch—broccoli bliss★

Mid-afternoon—green leathers★

Dinner—tempura★ and baby leaf spinach
with lentil sprouts and sweet chili sauce★

DAY EIGHT

Breakfast—cereal★

Mid-morning—2 super sweeties★

Lunch—fantastic fennel soup★

Mid-afternoon—sweet potato chips★ and date chutney★

Dinner—big plate mixed salad leaves and olives
dressed with avo pesto★

DAY NINE

Breakfast—breakfast pudding★

Mid-morning—fresh juice made with 4 sticks celery
and 1 apple

Lunch—porcini mushrooms and pesto★

Mid-afternoon—2 carrot cakes★

Dinner—fattoush★ and zucchini fries★

DAY TEN

Breakfast—cereal★

Mid-morning—seasonal fresh fruit

Lunch—"my favorite things"★

Mid-afternoon—1 chocolate brownie★

Dinner—pizza peppers★

DAY ELEVEN

Breakfast—"can't beta it"*

Mid-morning—2 crunchy quinoa crackers*

Lunch—Mediterranean stuffed tomatoes*

Mid-afternoon—salad bar*

Dinner—sweet potato satay* and simple salad*

DAY TWELVE

Breakfast—fresh juice made with 2 sticks celery,
2 carrots, and $\frac{1}{2}$ inch ginger

Mid-morning—2 flapjacks*

Lunch—nori rolls stuffed with hemp seed hummus*,
lettuce leaves, and alfalfa sprouts

Mid-afternoon—2 maca balls*

Dinner—sweetheart salad*

DAY THIRTEEN

Breakfast—rye bread* with jam*

Mid-morning—fresh juice made with 2 carrots,
1 apple, and 2 sticks celery

Lunch—cabbage medley*

Mid-afternoon—2 Lisa's raw Indian bars*

Dinner—parsnip rice* and "eat more greens"*

DAY FOURTEEN

Breakfast—best ever chocolate pudding*

Mid-morning—2 apple cashew cookies*

Lunch—oakleaf lettuce with pineapple dressing*

Mid-afternoon—plantain chips*

Dinner—Thai red curry*

Sprouting

here are many different sprouting gadgets on the market that you may choose to invest in, but personally I have always stuck with the old-fashioned jam-jar method. I use a quart-size glass jar for smaller quantities of sprouts. If I am doing large amounts, for example, a batch of buckwheat for dehydrating, I use a large Pyrex, ceramic, or glass bowl. Most sprouts simply need soaking in the purest water available, then rinsing once a day. In very hot weather you may need to rinse twice a day to prevent them going bad. I rinse mine by filling the receptacle they are in with pure water, swishing them around with my hands, then draining them off in a sieve.

Sprouts are an amazing food for several reasons. They are the ultimate in fresh food, so you know exactly how they have been grown and that they are still full of their life force! Sprouting increases the nutritional content drastically: proteins, minerals, vitamins, and enzymes increase and become more bioavailable. When you sprout grains, the starches that many people are intolerant to are converted into natural sugars, so most people who have a gluten problem are fine with sprouted wheat, spelt, rye, and oats. Finally, sprouting is incredibly economical as the raw seeds, beans, and grains cost pennies, and you can produce huge platefuls of sprouts for next to nothing.

The following are the sprouts that are commonly used throughout this book.

Aduki, mung, green lentil, brown lentil: soak 2 oz/60 g for 8–12 hours, sprout 3–5 days. These are among the easiest things to sprout. You can use them individually or make a mix and sprout them in the same jar together.

Alfalfa: soak 1–2 tbsp for 4–8 hours, sprout 7 days. This is a raw staple; a small amount of seeds makes a massive amount of sprouts.

Buckwheat: soak 5 oz/150 g for 5 hours, sprout 3 days. Buckwheat needs careful attention as it has a tendency to go slimy. Give the seeds a good rinse before soaking and another after. Don't soak for more than 5 hours. You get better results if you rinse twice a day.

Chickpea: soak 5 oz/150 g for 8–12 hours, sprout 3 days. Sprouting chickpeas is easy to do; don't let the tails get longer than the bean or they will taste woody.

Quinoa: soak 4 oz/120 g for 4–8 hours, sprout 3–5 days. Quinoa is quite tricky to sprout and needs lots of attention. Rinse twice a day.

Sunflower: soak 2 oz/60 g for 4–8 hours, sprout 1–3 days. Don't over sprout these or they taste bitter.

Wheat, spelt, oats, and rye: soak 3 oz/90 g for 8–12 hours, sprout 3–5 days. Sprouted grains are used for making breads, or for a filling. It's also a tasty and nutritious addition to salads.

Kitchen Notes

*T*he availability of raw food ingredients is growing steadily. It's very exciting to see all these new, previously unheard-of products come onto the market. Be adventurous and you will be astounded at the endless amount of new meals you can come up with.

Blenders

I have a Vita-Mix, and where I say "blender" in a recipe, that's what I've used. The Vita-Mix is an amazing machine, and revolutionized what I can do in the kitchen. It is basically a very high-powered blender, capable of blending just about anything. It also does a good job of grinding nuts, seeds, grains, beans, and so on. However, it is very expensive (at the time of printing, it retails for between about $350 to $600). It's a great investment, if you can afford it, and invaluable for easy and efficient raw food preparation. I haven't tested these recipes with a standard blender, but I know that your average machine would find some of the combinations hard work. If things aren't churning up nicely for you, try putting your mixture in the food processor with the S-blade in. Sometimes this on its own will do the trick, but for a smoother finish, put the mixture back in the blender and it should be able to handle it better. You can also try using a hand-held blender. These can be more efficient at achieving a thorough blending when a standard blender just isn't up to it.

Carob, mesquite, and lúcuma

Look for organic or wildcrafted raw carob powder. You can also buy whole carob pods, which make a delicious, healthy sweet snack. There are some nice carob bars on the market, including ones that are wheat-free, sugar-free, dairy-free, hydrogenated fat-free, as well as actually tasting good. We use carob flakes, which are wonderful for sprinkling as a garnish, or in cookie mixtures.

Mesquite is another powdered sweetener that also comes from a pod. The powder is ground from the seed pods of the mesquite, or algorroba, plant. It is from the same family as carob. Lúcuma is a powdered Peruvian fruit that has a wonderful shortbread flavor. You can substitute mesquite or lúcuma for carob in any recipe, or try using them in combination.

Dates and dried fruit

I love fresh dates; they're one of my preferred methods of sweetening a dish. Dates are so nutritious that in the desert, people survive for long periods on a diet of little else but dates and camel milk! The best ones are the Iranian dates, which aren't too expensive and are raw and fresh. If you can get them, I really recommend fresh dates over dried dates. Dried dates have usually been heat treated and aren't so nutritionally potent. If you are using dried dates in a recipe, always soak them for 20 minutes to 1 hour first. Drink the soaking water afterwards, it's yummy.

Most dried fruit is heated to various degrees and is best eaten sparingly because of its high sugar content. Buy only dried fruits that are unsulfured and have no added vegetable oils or sugar coatings.

Dehydrators

Basically a box with a fan and heating element, dehydrators are like a raw oven, heating food at very low temperatures to preserve the nutritional status and enzymatic activity. The most popular dehydrator is the Excalibur because the trays are a good size and easily accessible, and it has a variable temperature control. There are some cheaper ones around but they are not so user-friendly.

Some dehydrators have variable temperature controls, and some do not. We have not given any temperatures in this book: the standard temperature for dehydrating raw foods is 100°F/38°C.

Dried tomatoes

I generally make my own dried tomatoes by blending some fresh in a jug and then drying them in the dehydrator until they're crispy. It doesn't take long, and it's so much cheaper than buying shop ones, which often have salt or preservatives added. If you don't have a dehydrator, look for the ones that come dry in packets rather than the ones in jars covered in oil, as these are far more economical. Soak shop-bought ones in water for at least 20 minutes, up to an hour, before you use them.

Grain coffee

There are many different brands of grain coffee on the market, using grains such as barley. They are not raw, but when used in combination with carob powder in a recipe, produce a wonderful deep chocolately taste.

Juicers

With most juicers it is generally a case of you get what you pay for. Standard centrifugal juicers might seem like a good option when you are starting out, but they have a number of drawbacks. They can be difficult to clean, and with the cheaper models you don't always get a lot of juice out of them. Gear juicers are a better investment because they produce more juice and have extended warranties so will last you longer. Twin-gear juicers are the tops for making green juices out of vegetables like celery, cucumber, and leafy greens. Single-gear juicers juice fruits and vegetables efficiently and are the easiest to clean. Another advantage to gear juicers is that they can also be used with a homogenizing plate to make purees and nut butters. There are many different models of juicer available, costing up to around $600; shop around, and see which one will suit your needs and your pocketbook.

Kitchen scale

A standard kitchen scale is needed to make the recipes in this book. Dry ingredients are listed by weight (measurements given in both ounces and grams).

Lecithin granules

Derived from soya, lecithin helps with the emulsification of fats, so it is a good supplement to take with flax oil to aid the liver in absorption. It is also rich in phosphatidyl-choline, a good brain food. Lecithin granules have a pleasant, almost cheesy flavor and are another simple and easy ingredient to sprinkle on your salads.

Psyllium husk powder

Psyllium is a root similar to plantain. The husks are sold in pharmacies and whole food stores as a digestive aid. When soaked in water, they swell up and absorb the water, creating a sort of jelly, which acts as an intestinal broom. In raw food cuisine they act as an effective, healthy, animal-free gelling agent. I prefer to use powdered husks as they give a smoother, less grainy result.

Nuts and seeds

Nuts are best used in moderation. For a start, most of the packaged nuts have been heat treated to varying degrees—cashews are guaranteed not to be raw, with the exception of Sunfood ones. But nuts are quite hard work for the body to deal with, and if you eat too many they can leave you feeling sluggish and heavy. Consume large amounts on a regular basis (a common pitfall for raw food beginners) and you're going to congest your liver and make yourself sick. Have a shot of wheatgrass—if you feel sick, chances are you need to stay off the nuts for a while. As a general rule eat no more nuts in a day than you can hold in one fist.

Seeds are much gentler on the body than nuts, and more nutritionally dynamic. Sesame, pumpkin, sunflower, and hemp are the main four. I generally try and soak my nuts and seeds first before I use them—if you forget, it's not the end of the world, but it's a good habit to get into on a regular basis. On average, seeds need 4–8 hours, nuts 8–12 hours (because they're bigger). But even if you've only got 20 minutes, that's better than nothing. Soaking releases the enzyme inhibitors, making them more digestible and friendlier to the liver. And of course, it also makes them bigger as they swell up and absorb the water, so you're also getting more for your money.

Nut and seed butters

Raw nut and seed butters are becoming easier and easier to find. Now there is a wide range available, including raw tahini and white almond butter (indispensable as a base for sauces and dressings, as well as a spread for crackers and breads), pistachio, black sesame, cashew, hazelnut, and sunflower, hemp, and pumpkin seed butter. They aren't cheap, but are very high quality and so heavenly they are well worth the expense. Use them sparingly. Even raw nut butters are very congesting and should be eaten as treats, not by the spoon (although we've all done it!). Steer clear of nuts or seeds that have been roasted, making them difficult to digest, more mucus forming, and hard work for the liver.

Nutritional yeast flakes

These are not a raw product, but they are rich in B vitamins and a delicious addition to raw savory foods when used minimally, and favored commonly for their cheesy taste. The yeast in the flakes is inactive, so they are suitable for use by people who have a yeast intolerance.

Oats

Finding raw oats can be difficult. Oats go rancid easily, so they are commonly steamed to stabilize them; without this treatment they would only be able to sit on shop shelves for weeks rather than years. Ask the source whether the oats are truly raw and not steamed. Look for fresh oat groats and rolled oats. Oat groats are the whole oats that need to be soaked and sprouted before use. Rolled oats have been flaked and can be soaked first and used for oatmeal and flapjacks or ground into flour for raw cakes and pastries.

Oils

My preferred oils are coconut, flax, hemp, and olive oil. Coconut oil is a monounsaturated fat, which health experts are starting to believe is essential in the diet because of the essential fatty acids it contains, mainly lauric acid. Coconut oil is the only fat that is not metabolized by the liver, and is a superb source of energy. It is antimicrobial, antiviral, and balances the metabolism. Flax oil is the highest dietary source of the omega-3 essential fatty acids, which is the one Western diets mostly lack. Hemp oil is the only food that is the perfect balance of omegas 3, 6, and 9. They have very different but equally delicious flavors: flax is buttery, hemp is nuttier. When buying oils, look for those in dark glass bottles—with the exception of coconut oil, which is very stable, oils are sensitive to both heat and light. If an olive oil states it is from the first cold pressing, this should guarantee that it is raw. Olive oil is a great liver cleanser.

Olives

Are they raw or aren't they? Guaranteed raw olives are available in the United States. However, be aware that most olives have been heat treated. Steer clear of olives in brine and olives in tins, which are generally pasteurized. Pitted olives, too, are more likely to have been through intensive heat.

Sauerkraut

Fermented cabbage usually made with sea salt and juniper berries, sauerkraut is wonderful for the digestion because of its high enzymatic activity and the friendly bacteria it contains. It is a good source of vitamin C and helps strengthen the immune system. Most sauerkraut is heat treated; look for unpasteurized sauerkraut.

Seagreens

One of my very favorite ingredients, Seagreens is a wild wrack seaweed granule that has a complete nutritional profile, that is, it contains all the vitamins and minerals the body needs. It adds texture, flavor, and nutrition to just about any savory dish you can think of. It is expensive, but you only need a little—1 teaspoon per serving is ample.

Sea vegetables

Sea vegetables, as the most mineral-rich foods found in nature, deserve to be a staple part of everybody's diet. Dulse, a purple sea vegetable, is our firm favorite (I can eat a whole packet in one sitting!); it just needs a light rinsing under the tap, and is a wonderful source of calcium. Arame is stringy, needs soaking for 20 minutes, and is also popular because of its mild taste—very good with grated vegetables. Hijiki is similar to arame, but slightly fatter, with a more intense flavor, and needs soaking for up to an hour, in which time it will triple or even quadruple in size. Wakame is green and leathery, and must be soaked for 10 minutes before adding to salads. Nori sheets are an essential item in the raw food pantry for making nori rolls, the raw fooders' sandwich. The light green sheets have been toasted so are not raw; search for dark green ones. Nori flakes and powdered sea vegetables such as dulse, sea lettuce, and nori are perfect for using as a salad or soup garnish. Sea spaghetti is another favorite; it has an outstanding flavor, and you can simply stir some into a creamy sauce for a raw tagliatelle. Then there's kelp, a powdered sea vegetable, which is amazingly rich in minerals, especially iodine. We eat it every day; adults only need $\frac{1}{2}$–1 teaspoon a day, so you can add it to most dishes and barely notice the fishy flavor.

Shop for raw sea vegetable products, which of course are ideal. However, some varieties are heated at over 100°F. I think sea vegetables are such an important part of the diet that it is better to eat them even though they have been heat treated than not at all. Some brands are not heat treated but are preserved in sea salt. They need thorough rinsing before use but are very fresh and taste like they have come straight off the seashore!

Sweeteners

People often ask me what I use as a sweetener: there is really only one good raw alternative, and that is agave nectar, which comes from a Mexican cactus plant, has a low glycemic index, and tastes gorgeous—similar to maple syrup. Also available is yacon syrup, which is made from the Peruvian yacon root, and contains only fructoligosaccharides, a sugar that is not absorbed by the body. It has a malty flavor and is good to use as a spread or topping. However, if you are unwilling to shell out for these on a daily basis, there are plenty of alternatives on the whole food market, which may not be raw but are relatively healthful. You can buy agave syrup that is not raw, but less than half the price. Then there's apple concentrate or date syrup, which come from natural fruit sources; molasses, rich in essential minerals; and maple syrup. Any of these are acceptable if you're not strict about raw, and not having them in large amounts. Stevia is an herb that comes in powdered or liquid form. It is incredibly sweet (300 times sweeter than sugar) so you only need a tiny amount. It can be hard to get it right with stevia: too much and the taste is like strong licorice, not enough and your dish will lack sweetness. It is illegal to sell stevia as a sweetener in the United States and the United Kingdom, and most people in the health food industry believe this is due to pressure from the sugar manufacturers, rather than any proven health risks.

Tamari, shoyu, miso, liquid aminos, hemp sauce, Himalayan crystal salt

These are seasonings that we use to add a salty element to our recipes, and bring out the flavors of a dish. They are very strong, so use sparingly—the less, the better. Look out for miso that is unpasteurized, and with a low sodium content if possible. Although miso is not a raw food, it is a living food; due to the fermentation process it contains living enzymes. The original liquid aminos is made by Bragg. Paul Bragg was a raw food pioneer, and this product used to be very popular, but there is some controversy over it now because it contains hydrolyzed vegetable protein, and has naturally occurring MSG. My personal view is that a heavily processed product like this is never going to be good if you consume it by the tablespoon, but a dash on a salad will liven it up without causing the body any undue harm. Hemp sauce has a similar taste to liquid aminos, and is made with fermented hemp seeds and sea salt. It makes a good stock substitute in sauces and gravies. Himalayan crystal salt is an amazing pink salt found in one of the purest places on earth. Rich in minerals, it also aids absorption, and I love to add a pinch to savory or sweet dishes. You can also use crystal sea salt if you prefer.

Vanilla

Pods are the freshest and most flavorful option for whizzing up in your creams, ice creams, and sweets. If you are not using your blender, you can slit open the pod with a knife and scrape out the seeds to add to your recipe. Vanilla pods must be stored in an airtight container to preserve their taste and aroma. If you haven't got vanilla pods, vanilla extract is the next best option. This is not raw, and is preserved in alcohol, but it is pure vanilla. Steer clear of vanilla essence, which is a pale imitation of the real thing.

Vegetables

Where the recipe states "2 carrots" or "1 onion," this is taken to mean one average-sized vegetable. Please don't be afraid to play around with the amounts and adjust them accordingly. For instance, if your carrots are very large, and the recipe calls for two, perhaps it is better to just use one and a half; conversely, if your onions are very small, and the recipe asks for a half, better to use a whole one. One of the beauties of raw food preparation is that it is very hard to go wrong—it is not like traditional cookery where if your eggs are not whisked enough or your sauce not hot enough, disastrous results may befall you. Rather, be intuitive with your recipes, and the dish will taste wonderfully different every time.

Try and buy seasonally and locally whenever you can; it's best not to go chasing after ingredients that have been flown halfway across the world, especially when homegrown produce tastes so much better. Organic is preferable but not always the best option; I would argue that when it comes to flavor and nutrition, it's better to buy a local apple that is not certified organic than an organic one from the other side of the world. If the vegetable or fruit you are after is not in season locally, see if you can source an alternative that is. When buying salad greens look for minimal packaging; not only is all that plastic bad for the environment, it is affecting the quality of the produce too.

Vinegar

A good-quality, unpasteurized apple cider vinegar should be raw. We also occasionally use rice vinegar and balsamic vinegar, which are not raw. Other alternatives include lemon juice and lime juice.

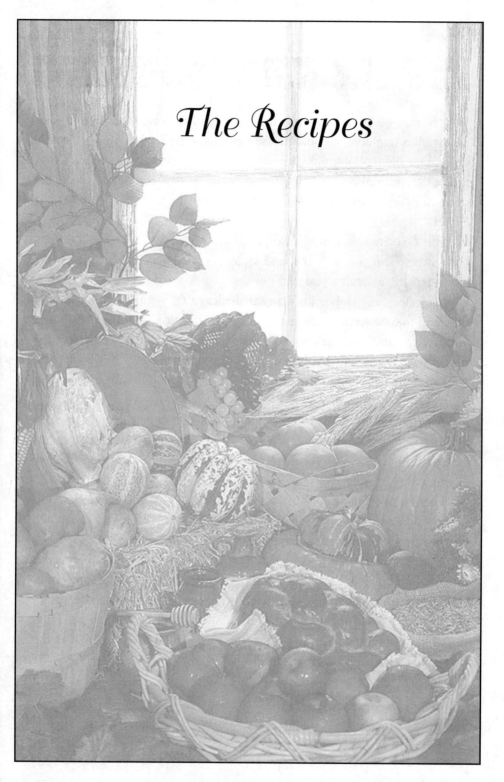

The Recipes

DIPS

Why so many dips? They really are a staple of the raw food diet, like the sandwich is to a conventional diet. Endlessly versatile, they turn a humble carrot into a feast. We usually have dips every day, either for lunch or tea. A recipe can be simply tweaked to create a whole new taste experience; the same dip can be used in different ways to create an amazing variety of dishes.

Our favorite vegetables for dipping are carrot sticks, broccoli florets, baby sweet corn, sugar snaps, and sweet potato (peel and cut into sticks like carrot). But really, you can use anything—mushrooms, cauliflower, pepper, celery, cucumber, anything at all. Serve a selection with one or two dips and maybe some chips made in the dehydrator (see page 168), and you have a quick and delicious light meal or snack. Dips are perfect for parties, easy to do when you're catering for large numbers of people, and very attractive, if you fan the different-colored vegetables out in a serving dish.

Another raw staple is roll-ups made with nori sheets. Spread the dip on the sheet, sprinkle with a few sprouts and some finely chopped vegetables, and roll up. You can try them with lettuce leaves, cabbage, or Chinese leaf too.

Finally, you can add a little water, thin them out, and make rich and interesting dressings for your salads. Just mix some green leaf in a bowl, and hey presto! A gourmet dinner in minutes.

You're also allowed to eat them with a packet of chips! Then you can indulge your cravings and get some super-nutrition in you at the same time.

Another tip: dehydrate your leftovers. Spread thinly on a sheet and, when they're dried through, store in an airtight tub in the fridge. Then crumble onto your salad for a bit of texture. Dehydrating intensifies the flavors to create delicious raw "croutons."

HEMP SEED HUMMUS

Blender

10 minutes (4–8 hours soaking)

Serves 4 to 6

This was our favorite dip for a long time. One tablespoon of sesame seeds contains eight times as much calcium as a cup of cow's milk, so it's great for growing children, and the hemp seeds ensure they get a good dose of those essential fatty acids. It's full of protein, but not too dense.

7 oz/200 g sesame seeds, soaked 4–8 hours

2 oz/60 ml hemp seeds, soaked 4–8 hours

1 lemon, juiced

1 tbsp olive oil

1 clove garlic

$\frac{1}{2}$ tsp Himalayan crystal salt

8 fl oz/250 ml water

Drain the sesame seeds and hemp seeds. Put everything in the blender together, and blend to make a creamy paste. The sesame seeds will break down completely, although you'll be left with black specks in the mixture from the hemp seeds, which crack open and release their beautiful rich oils. Keep in the fridge and eat within five days.

Did you know that George Washington was a hemp farmer, and the Declaration of Independence was written on hemp paper?

REUBEN'S GUACAMOLE DIP

Blender

5 minutes

Serves 4

My boys have always been fussy about avocados. Getting one that is a little overripe puts them off eating them. They insisted that they wouldn't eat guacamole, but I adore it. So I took their favorite dip, combined the two, and hey presto, something we all love.

1 lemon

1 large avocado

1 large tomato

2 tbsp tahini

1 tsp miso

1 tbsp nutritional yeast flakes

1 tsp kelp powder

Juice the lemon, and add the juice to the blender. Peel and pit the avocado, and add the flesh to the blender. Quarter the tomato, and add it into the blender with all the remaining ingredients. Blend to a cream. Serve with crudités. For a quick snack, spread some on a romaine lettuce leaf, add some alfalfa, roll up, and munch.

If you're into super foods, sprinkle some raw cacao nibs or bee pollen into your guacamole for an extra buzz.

RED PEPPER KETCHUP

Blender

10 minutes

Serves 4

*Wow! Much better than the tomato version, and healthier too.
Red peppers have a really high water content: if you blend them up,
they turn surprisingly liquid. Alternatively, use yellow peppers
for a golden ketchup.*

2 oz/60 g dried tomatoes (see page 171)

3 red peppers

4 dates

$\frac{1}{4}$ onion

1 tbsp apple cider vinegar

If you're using shop-bought dried tomatoes, you will need to soak them for up to an hour to soften them a bit first. Remove the stem and seeds, and chop the red peppers as small as you need to for your blender, then pop them in. Pit the dates, peel the onion, and add them in with the vinegar and tomatoes. Blend the whole lot together. The resulting blend should be the same consistency as ketchup—dollopy. Good with burgers, or just as a dip with crudités.

*Tomatoes are highly acidic, and avoided both by followers
of macrobiotics and Hippocrates practitioners.*

CARROT KETCHUP

Blender

10 minutes

Serves 4

Another alternative to tomato ketchup, carrots have a lovely fruity flavor when pureed into a dip.

2 oz/60 g dried tomatoes (see page 171)

4 carrots

4 dates, pitted

$\frac{1}{2}$ onion, peeled and chopped

1 tbsp apple cider vinegar

1 tsp miso

1 tsp kelp

4 fl oz/125 ml water

If you're using shop-bought sun-dried tomatoes, soak them for up to an hour first. Top and tail the carrots, and cut them into small enough pieces for your blender to be happy with them. Put all the ingredients in the blender and whiz up. If your carrots are big, you may need some more water, but not too much: you want it to have the thick consistency of traditional ketchup. Serve with burgers or spread on crackers.

Carrots are the richest vegetable source of vitamin A, the antioxidant that promotes good vision, hence the old wives' tale that carrots make you see in the dark.

ASIAN DIPPING SAUCE

Blender

5 minutes

Serves 4

This is like those red sauces you get with your Chinese or Thai spring rolls. It's quite runny, and wouldn't really work as a dip for crudités. But it's good with raw spring rolls or the tempura (see page 136). And it makes a super dressing on a salad of green leaves and sea vegetables.

3 tomatoes

1 red chili, seeded

1 clove garlic

1 tbsp tamari

1 tbsp agave nectar

1 tbsp sesame oil

Cut the tomatoes into quarters. Put everything in the blender and whiz until the tomatoes are fully pureed. Keep for an hour or two before serving, and it will thicken slightly.

It is a substance called capsaicin that gives chilies their heat: the more capsaicin the pepper contains, the hotter it is. Scotch bonnets and habaneros are the hottest varieties—we usually use the long, thin peppers commonly found in supermarkets.

SWEET ALMOND DIP

No equipment needed • 5 minutes • Serves 2

This is a favorite with kids: serve with veggies like carrot, cucumber, and broccoli and with any luck they will eat lots. It also makes a lovely dressing thinned with a little water.

1 tbsp agave nectar

2 tbsp almond butter

1 tbsp flax oil

1 tbsp nutritional yeast flakes

Put them all in a bowl and give them a good mix together with a spoon.

Almonds are rich in monounsaturated fats, which have been associated with reduced risk of heart disease, and have been shown to lower cholesterol.

PARSLEY DIP

Blender • 10 minutes (4–8 hours presoaking) • Serves 4

Lemons always add a tangy edge to any dip, and here they bring the flavors of the parsley to life. This is a very adult dip; children tend to find the parsley too overpowering, but it works in just about any way you choose to serve it—as a spread, a dip, in roll-ups, or as a dressing.

1 large bunch parsley

3 oz/90 g sesame seeds, soaked 4–8 hours

4 tbsp olive oil

2 lemons, juiced

1 tsp kelp

2 cloves garlic

Prepare the parsley, chopping it down so it will fit nicely in your blender. Drain the sesame seeds. Put everything in the blender and puree until smooth. If you don't have a high-speed blender, you may find this hard work. Chop the parsley really fine, and consider substituting half or all the sesame seeds for tahini.

There are two common varieties of parsley, flat leaf and curly.
Curly has a more intense flavor, and the flat leaf is more fragrant.
We like to use both, depending on how the mood takes us!

ZACHARY'S DIP

Blender • 10 minutes • Serves 4

When I was weaning my youngest son, this was his (and my) favorite lunch. Once he'd got past the baby food stage, I carried on making it as a dip. It's sweet without being too sugary, a lovely light dip, and with all that broccoli, very nutritious.

2 pears
2 small heads broccoli
1 tbsp flaxseed oil
2 tbsp tahini
2 tbsp nori flakes

Chop the pears and remove the cores and stems. Put them in the blender and they will easily turn to pulp. Add the broccoli, oil, and tahini, and blend again. Check that no broccoli heads have escaped the blades, and are hiding in the puree. Stir in the nori flakes by hand, or blend briefly. When you're sure it's all blended together, serve in lettuce wraps or nori rolls with lots of alfalfa.

Pears are a good source of the trace mineral copper—
an average pear contains 10 percent of the RDA.

CILANTRO CHUTNEY

Blender
5 minutes (4–8 hours soaking)
Serves 4; makes 1 jar

*Adapted from an authentic Indian recipe, this is a creamy, pungent
chutney, quite complex in flavor and slightly spicy. It goes well
with raw onion bhajis and is also lovely in lettuce wraps
teamed up with a heap of bean sprouts.*

1 large bunch cilantro
$\frac{1}{4}$ onion
1 chili, stem and seeds removed
1 lime, juiced
1 tsp garam masala
2 dates, pitted
1 tsp tamari
2 tbsp almonds, soaked 4–8 hours
4 fl oz/125 ml water

Loosely chop the cilantro. Put everything in the blender together and
blend to a thick puree.

*Along with basil and parsley, cilantro is a staple in our kitchen.
We often add a few sprigs to our vegetable juice,
or snip a few leaves into a salad to add an
exquisite something extra.*

DATE CHUTNEY

Blender

5 minutes

Serves 4

Gorgeous with burgers instead of ketchup.

5 oz/150 g pitted fresh dates

2 tbsp apple cider vinegar

1 tbsp sesame oil

$\frac{1}{4}$ inch piece root ginger

1 clove garlic

$\frac{1}{2}$ red chili

Put everything in the blender. It should turn to a cream more or less instantly if you're using good soft dates. Just make sure there are no pieces of garlic or chili left unprocessed!

Chili peppers have amazing healing properties. They are said to fight inflammation, reduce congestion, and boost immunity, even reduce the risk of cardiovascular disease.

LEMON PICKLE

Blender

5 minutes

Serves 4

*Preserved raw lemons go great in salads, but I love to eat them
in this addictive chutney. Beware though,
they are quite salty, so don't overdo it.*

1 red chili

4 fresh dates, pitted

$\frac{1}{2}$ inch root ginger

1 clove garlic

2 tbsp olive oil

7 oz/200 g preserved lemons

Remove and discard the stem and seeds of the chili. Put everything except
the lemons in the blender, and blend to a puree, being careful to make sure
there are no bits of chili or garlic left. If you're using a high-powered
blender, you can put the lemons in and blend them on a slow setting (3 or
4) to make sure they stay chunky. If not, you can process them in the food
processor, or chop them by hand, and then stir them back in. You want
them in chunks roughly the size of hazelnuts. Store in the fridge—it keeps
well. It goes great with burgers, as a dip for chips, or as a spicy salad
dressing.

*In mid-nineteenth century America, lemons were highly prized
for their ability to protect against scurvy, so much so
that they were sold for as much as $1 each!*

PÂTÉS AND SPREADS

Pâtés are always a winner stuffed in a pepper: just cut the pepper in half lengthways, seed it, and fill it with pâté. Cucumbers are good sliced crossways and spread with pâté to make little canapés. They're also easy to do spread on a lettuce leaf or nori sheet and rolled. Some of them are stiff enough that you can roll them into balls and serve them as little falafel-y things with a sauce. If you have a dehydrator, even better: pop the balls in for a few hours to make them crunchy and draw out the flavors. And of course, you can just use them as spreads for crackers and breads.

TAPENADE

Blender • 5 minutes (1 hour soaking) • Makes 1 small jar

Tapenade is a Mediterranean olive spread best made with pitted olives. Basically it's just an excuse to eat lots of olives, which are one of the best sources of healthy fats and protein around. This is a wonderfully rich, earthy dip, best spread sparingly on bread or crackers, or it makes a marvellous dressing on a pile of green leaves and sprouts.

1 oz/30 g dried tomatoes (see page 171)
3 oz/90 g pitted olives
1 tbsp olive oil
1 tsp vinegar
1 clove garlic, crushed

If you are using shop-bought dried tomatoes, you will need to soak them for up to an hour first. Unless you have a high-powered blender, you may find your food processor works better for this recipe. Just pop all the ingredients in, and blitz until completely pureed, with no bits of tomato left visible.

There is an olive tree in Croatia that has been determined by tree ring analysis to be nearly 2,000 years old, and is still producing fruit. I would love to try some of those olives!

OLIVE PÂTÉ

Blender

10 minutes

Serves 4

This is like a less rich version of the previous tapenade recipe, so you can
be more liberal with it. Try it on crackers or in roll-ups.

2 tomatoes

1 stick celery

1 sprig parsley

3 oz/90 g olives

$\frac{1}{2}$ red chili, seeded

2 tbsp dulse

1 tbsp olive oil

Quarter the tomatoes, and chop the celery and parsley down a little. Put
everything in the blender and process until smooth.

Olives are one of the best dietary sources of vitamin E,
the fat-soluble antioxidant. They are also rich in
monounsaturated fats, and it is this combination
that makes them exceptional nutritionally.

CASHEW CREAM CHEESE

Blender

5 minutes (8–12 hours presoaking)

Serves 4

This is lush, a good one to serve to non-raw fooders, it's so irresistible. If you're feeling extravagant, you can make it with macadamias or pine nuts for a real gourmet treat.

4 oz/120 g cashews, presoaked 8–12 hours

1 lemon, juiced

1 tsp miso

$\frac{1}{4}$ onion

8 fl oz/250 ml water

1 bunch chives

Put all your ingredients, apart from the chives, in the blender and keep it on for a good few minutes. Snip the chives into tiny pieces, as small as you can, with scissors, and then stir them in by hand. Cashews have a habit of hiding in the mix as little chunks unless you blend really thoroughly. If you store the spread in a jar in the fridge, it will thicken further.

Cashews are generally heat treated because the inside of the shell contains a caustic resin used to make insecticides! They are steamed at high temperatures to remove the nut from the shell without the resin. You can buy really raw cashews from online raw food stores.

HAPPY PÂTÉ

Blender

5 minutes (8–12 hours presoaking)

Serves 8; makes 2 jars

*This is one of my favorites. It's a really vibrant, fruity combination,
especially popular with children due to its natural sweetness.*

$\frac{1}{2}$ red pepper

2 carrots

1 tomato

2 oz/60 g almonds, presoaked 8–12 hours

2 dates, pitted

1 lemon, juiced

Prepare the pepper, carrots, and tomato and chop so they'll fit in your
blender. Add the remaining ingredients and blend. If it's too much for your
blender, add a little water or olive oil to help it along. Serve with green crudités such as broccoli, cucumber, and celery for a quick and easy snack
lunch. Store in the fridge, and eat within a few days.

*Almonds are actually seeds, which come from the fruit
of the almond tree. They are from the same family of
trees as apricots and peaches. I don't know why
we never eat almond fruit!*

Sunshine Pâté

Blender

5 minutes (8–12 hours presoaking)

Serves 8; makes 2 jars

This is like a more adult version of the previous recipe,
a little spicier and denser. It's a bit too thick to use as a dip,
but good for spreading in nori rolls or lettuce leaves.

2 carrots

2 tomatoes

1 yellow pepper

4 oz/120 g almonds, presoaked 8–12 hours

1 tsp tamari

1 lemon, juiced

1 tsp cumin powder

Prepare your carrots, tomatoes, and pepper by removing unwanted bits and chopping them small enough to fit into your blender easily. Pop them in (tip—put the tomatoes in the bottom because they liquidize easier and are not so likely to get stuck in the blades), and blend until smooth. Then add in the remaining ingredients, and keep blending until there are no lumps of nut left. Store in the fridge—it will only keep for a few days.

We always make sure to remove all the seeds from
our peppers. Although they are edible, they are bitter,
and contain no particular nutritional benefits.

WALNUT PÂTÉ

Blender

10 minutes (8–12 hours soaking)

Serves 4 to 6

*This is a lovely, dense, meaty pâté that makes a good stuffing
for peppers or nori rolls.*

2 sticks celery

1 red pepper

10 oz/300 g walnuts, soaked 8–12 hours

1 lemon, juiced

1 tbsp white miso

2 oz/60 g dried tomatoes (see page 171)

4 tbsp water

Chop the celery, remove the stem and seeds of the pepper, and chop. Put
everything in the blender and blend to a cream.

*Most people know by now that fish and flaxseeds are a good
source of the valuable omega-3 fatty acids, but did you know
that walnuts are also a great way to get these fats in your diet?
Twenty-five grams of walnuts contain about 90 percent
of the RDA.*

HAZELNUT AND APPLE PÂTÉ

Blender

5 minutes (8–12 hours soaking)

Serves 4; makes 1 large jar

This is a gorgeous, light, creamy pâté, good in nori rolls.

1 apple

1 tomato

1 stick celery

4 oz/120 g hazelnuts, soaked 8–12 hours

1 tbsp dried tomatoes (see page 171)

1 tsp white miso

2 tbsp olive oil

2 tbsp apple cider vinegar

Prepare the apple, tomato, and celery for your blender. Put everything in and blend to a thick puree.

Adding a little apple to any savory dish is a great way to lighten it up and create a contrast of flavors. Sprinkle grated apple into a salad, or blend half an apple into a soup or sauce.

PINE NUT PÂTÉ

Blender

5 minutes (4–8 hours soaking)

Makes I large jar

*This is very versatile—it makes a yummy dip or a rich dressing, it's great
in roll-ups, or it can be dehydrated for a very tasty salad garnish.*

4 oz/120 g pine nuts, soaked 4–8 hours

1 tbsp olive oil

1 small bunch basil

3 tomatoes, chopped

1 clove garlic

2 tsp white miso

Put everything in the blender. You shouldn't need any liquid, the tomatoes
will be enough. Blend for a few minutes until you have a light green cream.

*Pine nuts may be expensive, but they are very popular in raw
food cuisine for the creamy richness they impart to a dish, and
their exquisite fragrant taste. We buy ours in bulk and store
them in an airtight container in the dark so they keep well.*

DRESSINGS

Dressings can transform a simple salad into something amazing. Take a plateful of fresh leaves like arugula or corn salad (lamb's lettuce): add a spicy dressing to wake you up; a creamy dressing to soothe you; a fruity dressing to cheer you; a green dressing for cleansing; or an acidic dressing for a bit of zing. The resulting salad will be wildly different every time—who said raw food was boring? There's one here to suit your every mood.

My favorite simple dressing is flax oil, apple cider vinegar, Seagreens, and nutritional yeast flakes.

PESTO

Blender or food processor

10 minutes

Serves 4

I finally started making my own pesto, and it was a revelation. You need a large bunch of basil (if you're buying it in the supermarket, you may need two or three times what they consider a bunch), so it's not cheap. But the taste of pesto made with fresh basil is incomparable to the stuff that comes out of a jar. It's too rich to really use as a dip, but you could spread it on bread. Best as a dressing for salad.

1 large bunch basil, loosely chopped

2 oz/60 g pine nuts

2 tbsp nutritional yeast flakes

2 tbsp olive oil

1 tbsp agave nectar

1 tsp apple cider vinegar

2 cloves garlic

1 tsp tamari

Using your blender or food processor, put everything in and keep going until the basil is completely broken down and you have a thick gorgeous green goo.

Make some courgetti (that is, courgettes, or zucchini, done in the spiral slicer like spaghetti) and cover it in this, and hey pesto! You've got yourself a simply lovely dinner.

Avo Pesto

Blender

5 minutes

Serves 4

So quick, so easy, so yummy!

1 avocado

1 bunch basil

2 tbsp olive oil

2 lemons, juiced

2 cloves garlic

2 dates

1 tsp miso

Stone the avocado, scoop out the flesh, and put it in the blender. Cut the stems off the basil, chop loosely, and add to the blender with all the other ingredients. This is great on any salad, especially as a sort of coleslaw with grated vegetables like carrots and cabbage.

Adding avocado to salads can help with the absorption of both the antioxidants lycopene (found in tomatoes) and carotene (found in carrots). It is the monounsaturated fats in avocado that enhance the bioavailablity of these nutrients. This goes part way to explaining why raw fooders have a tendency to put avocado in everything!

CILANTRO PESTO

Blender

10 minutes

Serves 4

Hands up, who thought you could only make pesto with basil? OK, technically you are probably correct, but this version using fresh cilantro instead is just as delicious.

1 bunch cilantro

1 chili

4 tbsp olive oil

$2\frac{1}{2}$ oz/75 g Brazil nuts

2 limes, juiced

2 cloves garlic

2 dates

1 tsp tamari

Loosely chop the cilantro. Prepare the chili by removing the seeds and stem. Put everything in the blender and keep going until you have a thick cream. If your blender does not have a very strong motor, you may need to add a little water to help it turn.

Brazil nuts are one of the easiest nuts to make raw nut butter with. Put them in your blender or food processor and keep it on for a few minutes until it starts to get hot. If they're not runny already, leave the mixture to cool down for five minutes and repeat the process. Store fresh nut butters in the fridge to stop them from going rancid.

Coconut Satay

Blender

10 minutes

Serves 2

Fresh coconut is an incredible food, full of healthy fats like lauric acid,
an essential fatty acid found also in mothers' breast milk.
It combines well with dates, and this dressing manages
to be both refreshing and substantial.

4 oz/120 g coconut meat

2 tbsp olive oil

4 dates, pitted

$\frac{1}{2}$ chili, seeded

1 lemon, juiced

4 fl oz/125 ml water

Remove the flesh from the coconut shell. This involves a trick with a hammer and a chisel that I'm not very good at. Prize the flesh out of the nut with the chisel. Chop the coconut meat into small pieces and put in the blender with the other ingredients. If you have a high-powered blender, it will go gorgeously creamy. In a standard blender, the coconut won't break down completely, but you will still get a lovely mixture that works great as a dressing over some fresh green leaves. Eat within a day or two as fresh coconut goes rancid quickly.

To extract coconut flesh, find something to place the coconut
securely against, a doorstep is ideal. Whack the top with the
hammer about a third of the way down, rotate it slightly and
whack it again, and rotate and whack it again. Once you've
whacked it three times, the top should be easy to prize off.
Pour out the water and drink it—it's wonderful.

WALNUT DRESSING

Blender

5 minutes (12 hours presoaking)

Serves 4 to 6

*This is a very tasty, tangy dip to liven up your salad when you've only got
a few things left in the fridge, and are feeling devoid of inspiration.
Goes well on grated vegetables or a heap of leaves.*

5 oz/150 g walnuts, presoaked 8–12 hours

1 lemon, juiced

$\frac{1}{4}$ onion

1 tsp tamari

2 oz/60 g dried tomatoes (see page 171)

8 fl oz/250 ml water

Chuck everything in the blender and whiz away. If you have a dehydrator,
dry the leftover. It makes a gorgeous garnish, crumbled into a salad.

*Walnuts are good "brain food"! Not just because they look
like little brains, but because they are an excellent source of
omega-3 fatty acids, which promote mental clarity and focus.*

CREAMY CUCUMBER DRESSING

Blender

10 minutes (plus sprouting time)

Serves 4 to 6

*A creamy but surprisingly light dressing and all that cucumber
makes it very alkalinizing.*

1 cucumber

4 oz/120 g sprouted sunflower seeds (see Sprouting, page 49)

2 cloves garlic

1 lemon, juiced

1 tsp white miso

Chop the cucumber into pieces small enough for your blender to handle.
Blend everything up—it should whiz away quite easily. Pour over a pile of
green leaves. This is so good; you could even eat it as a soup.

*Sunflower seeds are one of the easiest seeds to sprout, a great
one to start with. They only take a day or two before they are at
their best—don't leave them too long or they will go brown.*

SWEET CHILI SAUCE

Blender

5 minutes

Serves 4; makes I small jar

You can buy a cooked version of this in Asian grocers and supermarkets. It's basically sugar and spice. The sweet taste makes the heat more palatable. It's traditionally used as a dipping sauce for spring rolls and barbecues, but we use it as a salad dressing.

16 dates, pitted

2 red chilies, seeded

3 cloves garlic

$\frac{1}{2}$ inch piece root ginger

2 limes, juiced

2 tbsp water

Prepare all your ingredients, and then put them in the blender with the water. Add more water if you want a runnier dressing: I like it nice and thick so it coats the salad well.

Ginger is very good for the digestion, soothing and calming to the intestines, which is why it is a popular home remedy for morning sickness during pregnancy.

PINEAPPLE DRESSING

Blender

5 minutes (10–20 minutes soaking)

Serves 4

This is a sharp, vibrant dressing. Take a plateful of arugula,
mix in some avocado and bean sprouts, toss it in this dressing,
and you have a meal fit for a king!

2 oz/60 g dried pineapple, soaked 10–20 minutes

$1/_4$ inch piece root ginger

1 clove garlic

1 lemon, juiced

2 tbsp sesame oil

2 tbsp water

Soak the pineapple in advance. When it is ready, drain it and add it to the
blender with all the other ingredients. Blend everything for a minute or
two, making sure there are no bits of ginger left floating.

Variations: replace the dried pineapple with dried papaya
or dried mango.

RED PEPPER DRESSING

Blender

5 minutes

Serves 4

Red peppers and lemons are just such a great combination.
Together they produce an unbelievably tangy fruitiness.
This dressing takes literally seconds to make, and yet can
transform a simple plate of leaves. Try it drizzled on arugula.

1 red pepper

2 tbsp olive oil

1 lemon, juiced

1 clove garlic

1 tbsp herbs de Provence

Remove the stem and seeds from the pepper. Chop it coarsely, and pop in the blender. Add the olive oil, lemon juice, and garlic and blend to a liquid. Stir in the herbs by hand, and serve immediately.

Herbs de Provence is an aromatic mix of dried herbs, usually
containing thyme, basil, marjoram, bay leaf, and rosemary.

SOUPS

Soups are about the easiest thing to make. All you need is a good blender, and you can have a great meal ready in minutes. Serve with some Essene (sprouted) bread or crackers and you've got a feast. Most raw soups don't really suit heating, but you can just gently warm them if you want something hot, especially in the winter. We use a porringer, which is a double saucepan that heats the water in the bottom pan, and so provides a more gentle heat for the top pan. Or you can put your soup in a Pyrex bowl in a saucepan of nearly boiling water. All the soups benefit from a sprinkling of dulse flakes, nori flakes, or nutritional yeast flakes and some alfalfa artfully strewn across the top.

CHICKPEA SOUP

Blender • 5 minutes • Serves 2

Creamy like hummus, this is a very filling soup. Don't over sprout chickpeas—the tails shouldn't be any longer than the beans or they start to taste a bit woody.

10 oz/300 g sprouted chickpeas (see Sprouting, page 49)

8 fl oz/250 ml carrot juice

3 tomatoes, chopped

1 tbsp tamari

4 tbsp olive oil

2 tbsp dulse, rinsed

2 tbsp dried tomatoes

2 cloves garlic

$1/_2$ red chili

16 fl oz/500 ml water

1 tbsp nori flakes

Chop the tomatoes. Chuck everything (except the nori flakes) in the blender and whiz away, until there's no point whizzing anymore—should take a couple of minutes. Pour into bowls and garnish with the nori.

Chickpeas are exceptionally nutritious, being an excellent source of protein and trace minerals, especially molybdenum and manganese.

FANTASTIC FENNEL SOUP

Blender

5 minutes

Serves 1

Fennel is one of my favorite vegetables, and makes a wonderfully light, simple, and refreshing soup. My other favorite fennel recipe is fennel and hijiki salad in pumpkin seed mayo (see page 115). I also juice fennel a lot; it's a lovely addition to a green juice.

6 tomatoes

1 avocado

1 head fennel

1 clove garlic

1 tbsp olive oil

1 tbsp tamari

Handful alfalfa sprouts

Prepare all the vegetables for the blender. Put the tomatoes in first because they are so liquid, they will be easier for the blades to start with. Reserve the alfalfa sprouts, and put everything else in the blender. Whiz for a minute, then pour into bowls and serve. Garnish with alfalfa sprouts.

Fennel also makes excellent chewing gum!
Chew on a stalk for extra-fresh breath.

BEETROOT SOUP

Blender

10 minutes

Serves 2

This is my all-time favorite soup. Sweet and spicy (if you're making it for children, just omit the chili). If your family isn't keen on beetroot, try them with this—they might be surprised.

2 beetroots

1 carrot

3 tomatoes

1 red chili

2 dates

2 tbsp olive oil

1 tsp tamari

8 fl oz/250 ml water

1 tbsp dulse flakes

1 tsp nutritional yeast flakes

1 tbsp pine nuts

Top, tail, and peel the beetroot. Chop into blender-friendly pieces. Top, tail, and chop the carrot, and cut the tomatoes into quarters. Seed the red chili. Pit the dates. Put all your prepared vegetables in the blender, along with the olive oil and tamari (tomatoes at the bottom to make it easy for your blender). Blend for a couple of minutes until you're satisfied there's no lumpy bits left. Pour into bowls and sprinkle with dulse, nutritional yeast, and pine nuts.

There is nothing quite like beetroot. Betacyanin is the pigment that stains your hands, chopping boards, and nice white tops . . . but, hey, it's also a powerful antioxidant, so that's OK.

SWEET CORN AND ALMOND SOUP

Blender

5 minutes (8–12 hours presoaking)

Serves 1

We try and eat seasonally in the main. This means that foods like sweet corn, which has a short season from July to September, become treats— delights that we anticipate all year round. In the sweet corn season, we eat it two or three times a week; it's great raw, straight off the cob. Then it's over, and we wait for next year's crop. Like Christmas or Easter treats, eating seasonally is fun!

1 cob sweet corn (approx. 4 oz/120 g)

1 stick celery

$\frac{1}{4}$ onion

1 oz/30 g almonds, soaked overnight

8 fl oz/250 ml water

1 tsp brown miso

1 tbsp olive oil

$\frac{1}{2}$ tbsp nori flakes

Strip the corn of its outer leaves, and remove the kernels from the cob by standing it over a bowl and slicing carefully downward with your knife, positioning the blade between the kernels and the cob. Roughly chop the celery and onion, and put them in the blender with the corn and the remaining ingredients (reserve the nori flakes). Blend for a good few minutes, making sure there are no bits of corn or almond left. Pour into bowls and sprinkle with nori flakes as garnish.

Corn comes in many colors, not just yellow, but blue, red, pink, black, and even purple. Purple corn is a rare and powerful antioxidant that is becoming a popular super food.

Autumn Leaves Soup

Blender

10 minutes (8–12 hours presoaking)

Serves 2

Reuben named this because of the colors, and the dulse garnish looks like leaves. But it's doubly appropriate because it's made with all the lovely root vegetables that start coming into season in the autumn. Use either parsnip or squash or sweet potato: they have quite distinctive flavors, and you will end up with a different soup every time.

1 lb/500 g root vegetables, such as butternut squash, sweet potato

2 large carrots

4 tomatoes

$\frac{1}{2}$ onion

2 tbsp almonds, soaked 8–12 hours

1 tbsp sesame oil

1 tbsp agave syrup

1 tbsp brown rice vinegar

1 tbsp tamari

1 tbsp Chinese 5 spice

2 tbsp dulse flakes

Prepare your vegetables so they'll fit happily in your blender. Squash and sweet potato need peeling. Put the tomatoes in the blender first because they liquify easily and will help everything else to turn over. Put everything in but the dulse flakes. Blend up to a puree; you need a high-powered blender to get a really good, creamy result. Pour into bowls and sprinkle with dulse flakes as garnish.

Chinese 5 spice is a great staple to have in your cupboard to add to dips and salad dressings. It's so called because it represents each of the five elements of Chinese medicine, and encompasses all of the five flavors—salty, sour, sweet, bitter, and pungent.

THAI PUMPKIN SOUP

Blender

15 minutes

Serves 2

*It's worth hunting down fresh herbs and spices from an Asian grocer
or well-stocked supermarket. You can buy more than you need,
and freeze the extra until the next time you are making a Thai recipe.
Failing that, powdered versions are acceptable, or you may
want to just use a ready-made Thai curry paste.*

1 medium-sized pumpkin

4 oz/120 g fresh coconut meat

2 sticks celery

$\frac{1}{2}$ inch piece root ginger

1 clove garlic

$\frac{1}{4}$ onion

1 red chili

2 dates

1 stick lemongrass

$\frac{3}{4}$ inch piece galangal

1 tbsp rice vinegar

1 tbsp tamari

2 tbsp sesame oil

Scoop the flesh out of the pumpkin. There's no easy way to do this, but if
you can get hold of a pumpkin scraper, they help. Put it in the blender. Prepare all the other ingredients for your blender, and pop them all in. Whiz
up for a few minutes to make a smooth, creamy soup.

*This is the perfect use for the pumpkin meat that is
discarded from making Halloween lanterns.*

PARSNIP SOUP

Blender

15 minutes

Serves 2

*This is gorgeously sweet and creamy,
perfect for a winter's lunch.*

2 parsnips

2 sticks celery

2 small carrots

1 avocado

2 dates, pitted

2 cloves garlic

1 tbsp rice vinegar

1 tsp miso

2 tbsp flaxseed oil

1 tbsp lecithin granules

20 fl oz/600 ml water

Prepare the vegetables to fit the blender. Top and tail the parsnips, and chop finely or they'll be hard to break down. Chop the celery and carrots. Halve the avocado, remove the pit, and cube the flesh. Put everything in the jug and blend to a thick puree.

*Lecithin is derived from non-GM (genetically modified) soy,
and comes in granular form. It is rich in phosphatidyl-choline,
which is important for brain development and assists
the body to absorb fats efficiently.*

SALADS

I was motivated to write my first book, *Eat Smart Eat Raw,* because so many people assumed being a raw foodist meant living on lettuce and bananas. "What do you actually eat?" was the most frequently asked question, and people couldn't believe it when I talked about Thai, burgers, noodles, and wraps. So here are even more super salad recipes, with barely a lettuce leaf in sight. While I was collecting the recipes for this book, I had been raw for about ten years and I was being pushed to find ever more inventive and creative ways of making original and interesting dinners. I explored new ingredients, and found simple and delicious ways to put them together. With two children, and another on the way, I wanted to make meals that would leave me and the family feeling full and nourished, but I didn't have the time or energy to spend long hours in the kitchen slaving over a dehydrator! Most of them are suitable either to be served individually as a meal in themselves, or if you want to liven things up a little, you can serve two smaller portions of complementary salad recipes together, or mix them with some of the recipes from the Savory Entrées section. Have a look at the Sample Menus on page 45 if you need more ideas.

CABBAGE MEDLEY

Food processor, blender • 10 minutes • Serves 4

Red cabbage contains more nutrients than white cabbage, for instance, at least six times the vitamin C. Sauerkraut is also a great source of vitamin C, as well as containing friendly bacteria, which are good for the digestion.

Avo pesto (see page 82)

14 oz/400 g red cabbage

14 oz/400 g green cabbage

8 oz/250 g sauerkraut

2 oz/60 g olives

2 oz/60 g mixed bean sprouts (see Sprouting, page 49)

Prepare the avocado pesto. Slice the red and green cabbage using the fine slicing plate on your food processor. Transfer to a mixing bowl. Add the sauerkraut, separating the strands out with a fork. Add the olives and bean sprouts. Using a fork or salad servers, toss the salad in the pesto, making sure all ingredients are evenly distributed.

This is really good served with parsnip rice (see page 103).

"CHICKEN" SALAD

Food processor

10 minutes

Serves 2

Try and eat an oyster mushroom whole, and it'll probably make you feel a bit sick, with its rich, earthy taste and spongy texture. But fine slice oyster mushrooms and they miraculously turn into tender white meat, similar to chicken, very succulent and not at all overpowering.

$^1\!/_2$ oz/15 g arame, soaked 10 minutes

2 oz/60 g dried tomatoes (see page 171)

2 bunches watercress

6 lettuce leaves

7 oz/200 g oyster mushrooms

2 oz/60 g mixed bean sprouts (see Sprouting, page 49)

2 oz/60 g pickled onions

2 cloves garlic, crushed

1 tbsp tahini

1 tbsp flax oil

1 tbsp apple cider vinegar

1 tsp white miso

1 tbsp Seagreens

1 tbsp water

Soak the arame. If you are using shop-bought dried tomatoes, you can halve the amount, and soak them in the same water. Using scissors, snip the watercress into bite-sized pieces, straight into the salad bowl. Shred the lettuce leaves and add them in. Fine slice the oyster mushrooms in a food processor or salad slicer, and add them to the mix, along with the bean sprouts and onions. In a small bowl, using a hand whisk, blend the remaining ingredients together to make a dressing. By now your arame should be ready—drain it and add it to the salad bowl with the tomatoes. Pour the dressing over the salad, toss, and serve immediately: watercress wilts quickly.

This is quite a substantial salad and would be enough on its own. If you want to add anything, some Lebanese cauliflower crackers (see page 159) would complement it nicely.

Mediterranean Salad

No equipment needed • 15 minutes • Serves 4

*This is a very simple salad to prepare, but if you get fresh, seasonal
ingredients it's a real winner. If you're not strictly raw, baby new
potatoes are a wonderful treat if you buy the first of the season.
Peas aren't raw either: unless you buy them in their pods and shell them
yourself, they are most certainly blanched. We use jars of organic peas.*

1 lb/500 g baby new potatoes (optional)

1 lb/500 g cherry tomatoes

1 cucumber

2 yellow peppers

12 leaves romaine lettuce

7 oz/200 g olives

7 oz/200 g green peas

4 tbsp olive oil

2 tbsp balsamic vinegar

1 tbsp nori flakes

Pinch sea salt

Pinch black pepper

If you are using potatoes, clean them, halve them, and put them in a pan
covered in water. Bring them to a boil, and simmer for 10–15 minutes.
Meanwhile, halve the tomatoes and pop in a large salad serving bowl.
Finely dice the cucumber, and add to the bowl. Fine slice the peppers and
lettuce in a food processor if you have one, and add to the bowl along with
all the remaining ingredients, including your new potatoes. Give everything
a good toss, so they are nicely covered in oil and vinegar. Serve immediately.

*Balsamic vinegar is not raw, but it has such a delicious flavor that
it is a very handy thing to keep in your cupboard for making a
plate of vegetables more interesting. When Reuben was about five,
one of his friends would come over to play frequently, and
always demand "lettuce and balsamic vinegar" for lunch!*

CURRIED OKRA

Blender

5 minutes

Serves 2

Okra is one of those foods people either love or hate; I am definitely in the former camp. When you cut it and either cook it or blend it up, it releases a sticky, glutinous substance and thickens the dish it is in.

6 tomatoes

2 tbsp dried tomatoes

2 tbsp olive oil

2 tsp curry powder

8 oz/250 g okra

Blend up everything but the okra. Chop the okra finely and add it in. If you have a Vita-Mix, blend it in on a 3 setting. The okra and tomatoes will amalgamate to produce an authentic Indian dish.

Okra, also known as lady's fingers, is not only used in Indian catering, but is popular in African and Middle Eastern cuisine.

FENNEL AND LEEK SALAD

Food processor

15 minutes (10 minutes presoaking)

Serves 2

Leeks are a wonderful addition to a raw dish, surprisingly mild and pleasant. I love the way the stems separate out into rings. Smaller ones are better, as they are sweeter and more delicate. You can use just about any dressing on this simple salad; a creamy choice such as avo pesto (page 82) works well. If you're in a hurry, just chuck on a splash of olive oil and a sprinkle of sea salt and ground pepper.

$\frac{1}{2}$ oz/15 g wakame, soaked 10 minutes

1 bulb fennel

1 leek

$\frac{1}{2}$ cucumber

1 oz/30 g bean sprouts (see Sprouting, page 49)

Any dressing (see Dressings, page 81)

Soak the wakame in advance. Using the fine-slicing blade on your food processor, slice the fennel, leek, and cucumber. Transfer to a mixing bowl. Add the bean sprouts and drained wakame. Mix evenly. Pour in your dressing, and toss. Serve immediately.

Look for good-quality sea vegetables in your whole foods or health food store. You can pick some up cheaper in Asian grocers, but the quality is nowhere near the same.

PARSNIP RICE

Food processor

10 minutes (8–12 hours soaking)

Serves 4

It was years before I realized that you could eat parsnips raw. Go on, try one, and take a bite. They have a distinctive sweet taste, but a woody texture that makes them hard work to chew, and not the sort of thing you'd nibble on like a carrot. But if you cut them into small enough bits, you can bypass this challenge and enjoy their unique flavor.
Also, check out the parsnip soup recipe on page 96.

$\frac{1}{2}$ oz/15 g wakame

4 parsnips

4 oz/120 g cashews, soaked 8–12 hours

2 tbsp sesame oil

1 tbsp rice vinegar

1 lemon, juiced

1 tbsp date syrup

1 tbsp tamari

Snip the wakame into tiny pieces with scissors. Soak in filtered water for 10 minutes while you prepare the other ingredients. Top and tail the parsnips, and chop them into chunks. Pop them in the food processor with the cashews, and process until they're about the size of rice grains. Transfer to the mixing bowl, and add the remaining ingredients along with the drained wakame. Give it all a good stir, and serve within 24 hours. (Store in the fridge if you don't serve immediately.)

If you've tried wakame and aren't a fan,
you could use dulse or sea spaghetti in this recipe instead.

SWEET POTATO SATAY

Food processor, blender
20 minutes (8-12 hours soaking)
Serves 4

Sweet potatoes are another of those vegetables that you wouldn't immediately think of eating raw. But they are surprisingly good, a bit like a cross between a carrot and an apple. You can peel them and cut them into sticks and serve them with a dip, or try them grated as in this recipe. The dates bring out the sweetness of the potatoes.

5 oz/150 g almonds, soaked 8–12 hours
2 oz/60 g pitted fresh dates
1 lemon, juiced
1 red chili, stem and seeds removed
4 tbsp water
1 tbsp tamari
2 sweet potatoes
2 oz/60 g fresh coconut pieces

To make the satay sauce, put the almonds, dates, lemon juice, chili, and water in the blender, and blend to a cream. Scrub the potatoes (you don't need to peel them) and grate them, using a fine grater. Put them in a mixing bowl. Grate the coconut pieces, and add them to the bowl. Pour the sauce over and mix thoroughly.

If you can't get fresh coconut, desiccated, chips, creamed, or even butter will do just fine.

Spicy Beetroot and Hemp Salad

Food processor

10 minutes

Serves 4

Beetroot is more commonly eaten cooked in the United States and the United Kingdom, but it is fantastic raw too, with a delicious sweetness that is complemented by the apple in this salad.

1 lb/500 g beetroot

2 apples

2 tbsp hemp seeds

2 tbsp hemp oil

1 tsp chili sauce

Top, tail, and peel the beetroot. Slice the apple into quarters and remove the core. Using a coarse grater, grate the beetroot and apple. Put them in a mixing bowl, with the remaining ingredients and toss.

Children like the natural sweetness of this dish, and the beetroot is a great source of iron, while they're getting lots of essential fatty acids in the hemp. Just omit the chili and add a dash of extra agave or raw honey.

PORCINI MUSHROOMS AND PESTO

No equipment needed

5 minutes (70 minutes soaking)

Serves 2

*Dried porcini mushrooms have a rich, deep earthy flavor that
when added to a salad can transform it from a humble lunch
into something fit for royalty.*

1 ½ oz/45 g dried porcini mushrooms

1 tsp olive oil

1 tsp tamari

1 tsp nutritional yeast flakes

2 tbsp hijiki

Pesto (see recipe page 81)

4 leaves lettuce

3 oz/90 g lamb's lettuce (mâche)

12 olives

Soak the porcini mushrooms in filtered water for 10 minutes. Drain, and marinate in olive oil, tamari, and nutritional yeast flakes for 1 hour. Soak the hijiki in filtered water for 30 minutes. If you haven't done so already, this would be a good time to prepare the pesto (or you can cheat, and use shop-bought pesto).

Once your pesto is prepared, and everything is soaked and ready, tear the lettuce into fine strips, and put in a serving bowl with the lamb's lettuce and olives. Add the drained hijiki and the mushrooms, which will have absorbed all the marinade. Spoon on the pesto, give it a good toss with the salad servers, and serve immediately.

*Porcinis are one of the most highly prized mushrooms
for their gourmet taste. They grow mainly in Europe
and are usually sold dried.*

ORIENTAL COLESLAW

Food processor

10 minutes

Serves 4

*This is like raw stir-fry! A good tip if you're craving some hot food is to
create a semi-raw stir-fry by cooking some sturdier vegetables, like onions
and cabbage, and then throwing some in at the end raw, like finely sliced
carrots and broccoli. This is a good way to trick your body into thinking
it's getting cooked food but still getting lots of raw goodies in there.*

2 tbsp arame

3 carrots

3 Jerusalem artichokes

1 small onion

4 oz/120 g sprouted chickpeas (see Sprouting, page 49)

$1/_2$ inch root ginger, minced

1 clove garlic, minced

2 tbsp sesame oil

1 tbsp date syrup

1 tbsp tamari

1 tbsp rice vinegar

Soak arame in filtered water for 10 minutes while you're preparing the vegetables. Top and tail the carrots and artichokes. Top, tail, and peel the
onion. Put them all through a coarse grater. Transfer to a mixing bowl and
spoon on the remaining ingredients. Drain the arame and add it in. Give it
a good mix around, and serve within a few hours.

*I love Jerusalem artichokes, but they are often overlooked.
Kind of like apple-flavored radishes, they are crisp and crunchy,
cleansing and refreshing, and make a welcome change to
carrots or cabbage in any sort of coleslaw dish.*

Simple Salad

No equipment needed • 5 minutes • Serves 1

This was a favorite family dinner for ages—simple but irresistible.
Serve with a slice of Essene (sprouted) bread and tahini
for the perfect quick but satisfying dinner.

3 leaves romaine lettuce

2 oz/60 g lamb's lettuce

2 tbsp sauerkraut

1 oz/30 g alfalfa sprouts

1 tbsp olives

1 tbsp seeds or nuts—whatever you favor

1 tbsp flax oil

1 tsp apple cider vinegar

2 tbsp dried sea vegetables

1 tbsp nutritional yeast flakes

1 tsp kelp powder

1 tsp lecithin granules

Wash the lettuces (we wash and dry them in a salad spinner) and shred very fine. Put in the salad bowl with everything else and give it a good mix round, so all the dried sea vegetables are evenly coating the lettuce. Serve immediately.

Lamb's lettuce is the family's favorite salad green.
It comes by many names—corn salad, lamb's leaf,
field salad, or sometimes mâche. It is sweet, tender,
and very easy to eat in huge quantities!

SATURDAY SALAD

No equipment needed • 15 minutes (1 hour soaking) • Serves 2

It used to be a Saturday tradition to sit together as a family and share a big meal. We used to call it "Saturday Dinner Party"; most often we would have this salad with some dips and chips. Then a few hours later, we would have a light supper, usually just pudding or cake. I love this salad, because you can really pig out on it, eat until you're full, and still feel wonderfully light and virtuous afterward.

1 oakleaf lettuce

1 avocado

1 small head broccoli

4 gherkins

1 oz/30 g hijiki, soaked 1 hour

2 tbsp curry crunch (see page 168)

1 oz/30 g alfalfa sprouts

2 tbsp flax oil

1 tbsp balsamic vinegar

1 tbsp Seagreens

1 tbsp lecithin granules

2 tbsp nutritional yeast flakes

Rinse and tear the lettuce, and pop it in a salad bowl. We use a salad spinner for lettuce to get it nice and dry. Halve the avocado, remove the pit, score the flesh into cubes, and scoop them out into the bowl. Chop the broccoli into small florets, put them in the bowl. Slice the gherkins thinly, and add them in with the hijiki, curry crunch, and alfalfa. Give it a good mix around, then add the remaining ingredients and toss. Serve immediately.

Red oakleaf is my favorite lettuce, but you can substitute whatever appeals. I very rarely go for the commonly found iceberg, baby gem, or round lettuces that more often than not seem a bit insipid. We like the more robust lollo rosso, radicchio, batavia, or good old romaine.

CURRIED PARSNIPS

Food processor, blender

10 minutes (8–12 hours marinating)

Serves 4

*Parsnips, with their natural sweetness, lend themselves surprisingly well
to salad. Eaten as they are, they are woody and hard work. But grate
and marinate them, as in this recipe, and you will be won over!*

4 parsnips

1 avocado

1 lemon, juiced

2 tsp cumin powder

1 tbsp garam masala

$\frac{1}{2}$ red chili pepper, seeds removed

Top and tail the parsnips. Grate them finely. Scoop the flesh out of the avocado. Put it in the blender along with the remaining ingredients, and blend to a puree, adding a little water if needed. Transfer the parsnips and dressing to a serving bowl, and toss. You can serve this salad right away if you wish, but if you have time, leave it in the fridge for at least a few hours, preferably a day, to allow the parsnips to tenderize.

*Grated parsnips are also delicious marinated in
avo pesto (see page 82).*

ZUCCHINI FRIES

Dehydrator

5 minutes (12 hours marinating, 8 hours dehydrating)

Serves 2

Potatoes were the last cooked food I stopped enjoying. It was years, maybe even a decade, before I could go past a chip shop in winter without lusting after some chips. Amazingly, the cravings stopped eventually, and now if I met you in a chip shop I would not even be tempted to sneak one off your plate! These are reminiscent of chips, or fries—greasy, covered in salt and vinegar, and, if you eat them straight out of the dehydrator, even warm.

1 lb/500 g (approx. 3) zucchini

1 tbsp balsamic vinegar

2 tbsp olive oil

1 tbsp tamari

2 tbsp dried sea vegetables

Slice your zucchini into fat, chunky french fries by topping and tailing, slicing them in half widthways, and then slicing each half lengthways into quarters. Put them in a shallow bowl or serving dish, pour over the vinegar, oil, and tamari, and toss in the sea vegetables. Marinate for 12 hours, stirring at regular intervals to make sure the zucchini is evenly coated. They should absorb most of the liquid. At the end of 12 hours, lift your fries separately onto the drying trays of your dehydrator. Any leftover marinade can be used as a salad dressing. Dry the fries for 6–8 hours. Eat warm straight from the dehydrator—they're not half as convincing as french fries when they're cold.

You say zucchini . . . ever look at a British or Australian website and wonder at some of the ingredients? Here's a quick rundown of some of the terms. Courgettes = zucchini, spring greens = collard greens, calabrese = broccoli, coriander = cilantro, aubergine = eggplant.

EAT MORE GREENS

Food processor • 10 minutes (10 minutes soaking) • Serves 2

This is a variation of one of my favorite recipes from Eat Smart
Eat Raw. *Here's a new twist on an old favorite, as they say.*

1 lb/500 g greens (such as kale, cavalo nero,
turnip greens, sprouting broccoli)

$^1/_2$ oz/15 g wakame, soaked 10 minutes

8 oz/250 g sauerkraut

1 large or 2 small avocados

1 tbsp Seagreens

2 tbsp nutritional yeast flakes

Chop the greens into manageable pieces and put them in the food processor. Blitz them until they're as chopped as they can be. Add in the drained
wakame and sauerkraut and process again, briefly, so they're mixed in.
Scoop the flesh out of the avocado and add that into the mix, along with
the Seagreens and yeast flakes. Process for a few minutes until there are no
lumps of avocado left. Serve immediately.

*With all the fantastic quality green vegetables available in
farmer's and whole foods markets, there's no excuse for them
not forming a central part of our diet. Although at first you
might find them a bit chewy eaten raw, you can mash them up
as in this recipe, make them softer by massaging olive oil into
the leaves, or juice them if you have a good-quality juicer.*

DAHL

Blender, food processor • 30 minutes (4–8 hours soaking,
plus sprouting time) • Serves 4

*Dahl is an Indian lentil soup, traditionally made with red split lentils. Split
lentils don't sprout, so we use brown, green, or Puy lentils. They are all easy
to sprout, and when mixed together look very pretty. This dish is a great way
to get people who aren't usually keen on bean sprouts to eat lots of them!*

1 lb/500 g mixed lentil sprouts (see Sprouting, page 49)

4 tbsp olive oil

1 tbsp tamari

1 tsp cumin

2 cloves garlic

3 oz/90 g sesame seeds, soaked 4–8 hours

2 lemons, juiced

1 small bunch cilantro

16 fl oz/500 ml water

1 red pepper

2 carrots

5 oz/150 g cauliflower

1 small head broccoli

In the blender, put the lentil sprouts, olive oil, tamari, cumin, garlic,
sesame seeds, lemon juice, cilantro, and water. Blend to a thick cream. This
is your dahl. (If you add less water, it makes a kind of lentil hummus you
can eat as a dip.) Next, assemble your vegetables and chop them roughly
into small pieces, about the size of cashew nuts. You can do this by hand,
using the S-blade on a food processor, or with your Vita-Mix on a slow setting. Transfer the dahl and the vegetables to a large bowl, and stir everything around with a spoon so the vegetables are evenly mixed in. Divide
between four bowls, and serve immediately.

*Sprouted lentils are an excellent source of raw protein, so this dish is
especially good for athletes, children, and breastfeeding moms.*

FATTOUSH

Blender

10 minutes

Serves 2

This is my version of the classic Lebanese salad. I love zaatar—it is worth
tracking down from a specialty grocer if you can. It's an aromatic mix
of thyme, sumac, and sesame seeds that the Lebanese believe
gives strength and calms the mind.

Small bunch mint

Small bunch parsley

2 lemons, juiced

4 tbsp olive oil

1 tbsp Liquid Aminos

1 tbsp zaatar

4 tomatoes

$\frac{1}{2}$ cucumber

2 bunches watercress

Make a pesto with the mint, parsley, lemon juice, olive oil, Liquid Aminos, and zaatar. Quarter the tomatoes and cube the cucumber. Chop the watercress. Mix all together.

Watercress is grown in shallow gravel beds and needs a
constant supply of fresh spring water—a mature bed can
consume as much as 5,000 gallons of water an hour! It takes
one to three months to grow, depending on the time of year.

FENNEL AND HIJIKI SALAD IN PUMPKIN SEED MAYO

Food processor, blender

15 minutes (4–8 hours soaking)

Serves 4

I adore this salad. Fennel is one of my favorite vegetables; with its
distinctive flavor, refreshing crispness, and unusual shape, you could
never accuse fennel of being boring. The pumpkin seed mayo makes
a gorgeous creamy contrast, so this salad manages to combine
a feeling of being virtuous and sinful at the same time.

14 oz/400 g white cabbage

1 bulb fennel

1 oz/30 g hijiki, soaked 1 hour

4 oz/120 g pumpkin seeds, soaked 4–8 hours

1 tbsp hemp oil

1 lemon, juiced

1 clove garlic

4 fl oz/125 ml water

Sea salt and black pepper to taste

Slice the cabbage and fennel using a fine slicer. Transfer to a mixing bowl
with the drained hijiki. Put the pumpkin seeds, hemp oil, lemon juice, garlic, and water in the blender and blend for a few minutes until you have a
thick cream. Spoon it over the vegetables—you will only need about two-
thirds of it, just enough to cover them, not drown them. Reserve the rest of
the mayo for another use, or dehydrate it. Serve immediately.

Pumpkin seeds are such a storehouse of nutrition, we try and
eat them every day, either on their own as a snack, in nut
butter, or blended into a dip or a sauce. As well as being one
of the richest dietary sources of zinc, they are an exceptionally
good source of the amino acid tryptophan, which raises
serotonin levels in the brain.

RED CABBAGE AND APPLE

Food processor, blender

10 minutes

Serves 2

*This is based on a German dish, traditionally made by braising the
red cabbage and apple, and popular at Christmas. But as you're
hopefully realizing by now, any recipe worth its sea salt works
just as well raw as it does heated!*

8 oz/250 g red cabbage

2 apples

1 tbsp vinegar

1 tbsp olive oil

1 tbsp raisins

Shred the red cabbage, and transfer to a mixing bowl. Blend the apples,
vinegar, and olive oil to a puree. Stir into the red cabbage with the raisins.
This salad can be left for a few hours or up to a day and the cabbage will
tenderize slightly in the apple.

*This is an unusual mix of flavors—bitter cabbage, sweet apples,
and sour vinegar—which combines to great effect.
If you like goji berries, you could use them as a
substitute for the raisins.*

MASHED PARSNIPS

Blender

5 minutes

Serves 2

This is my favorite way of eating raw parsnips, creamy and comforting, and so warming; you'll forget they're not cooked! You can dehydrate any leftovers to make parsnip chips.

1 lb/500 g parsnips

4 tbsp olive oil

4 fl oz/125 ml water

Sprinkle of sea salt

Chop the parsnips finely, add everything to the blender, and puree to a cream. This works best with either a high-speed blender or a hand blender. Serve immediately.

This works equally as well with celeriac instead of parsnip, or try half carrot and half parsnip.

CHRISTMAS COLESLAW

Food processor, blender

10 minutes (8 hours presoaking)

Serves 4

Is it possible to have Christmas dinner without Brussels sprouts?
Only if you're a spoilsport. In all honesty, Brussels sprouts aren't
great raw, a bit too crunchy and hard work for the jaws.
But grated in this salad as a replacement for cabbage,
they make a fantastic, fresh, and original coleslaw.

1 oz/30 g arame, soaked 10 minutes

2 carrots

1 apple

$\frac{1}{2}$ onion

7 oz/200 g Brussels sprouts

2 oz/60 g chestnuts (precooked from a tin or jar)

2 oz/60 g peas

4 oz/120 g cashews, soaked 8–12 hours

1 lemon, juiced

1 tsp white miso

Water

Soak the arame. Top and tail the carrots. Quarter the apple and remove the core. Finely grate the carrots, apple, onion, and Brussels sprouts. Transfer to a mixing bowl with some good-quality chestnuts, the peas, and arame. To make the mayonnaise, blend the cashews, lemon juice, miso, and water. Toss the vegetables in the mayonnaise. This salad will keep for a day or two, and the vegetables will soften and the flavors improve.

Brussels sprouts belong to the Brassica family of vegetables,
like cauliflower, cabbage, and broccoli, and contain
high amounts of the phytonutrient sulfur.

JANE'S CURRY

Food processor, blender

15 minutes

Serves 2

This was sent to me by a friend of a friend.
It's so easy to do, and really tasty.

2 avocados

2 lemons, juiced

2 tbsp sesame oil

1 tbsp curry powder

4 carrots

1 apple

3 oz/90 g fine green beans

1 red onion

2 stalks celery

1 red pepper

2 oz/60 g pine nuts

1 oz/30 g raisins

Start by making the curry sauce. Remove the flesh from the avocados and put it in the blender. Add the lemon juice, sesame oil, and curry powder, and blend to a cream. If it won't turn over, add a little water to get it to a creamy consistency. Next prepare your vegetables. Grate the carrots and apple and transfer to a mixing bowl. Fine slice the green beans, onion, celery, and red pepper, and add them to the bowl. Add the pine nuts, raisins, and avocado mixture and give it all a good stir. Serve immediately.

In Ayurvedic medicine, they recommend you rinse your mouth
with a tablespoon of raw sesame oil daily, to cleanse the whole
body and expel toxins and pathogens. They say it helps
to protect the body against colds and flus.

CREAMY CUCUMBER AND APPLE

Food processor, blender • 10 minutes • Serves 4

*The freshness of the cucumber and mint in this salad contrasts
exotically with the creamy sweet avocado dressing.*

1 cucumber

1 apple

4 oz/120 g sweet-corn kernels

1 bunch mint

1 avocado

4 fresh dates, pitted

1 lemon, juiced

2 tsp white miso

4 tbsp water

Top and tail the cucumber, and grate it using a coarse grater. Core the
apple and coarse grate that too. Put both in the mixing bowl, along with the
corn kernels. Remove the mint leaves from the stems, discard the stems,
and put the leaves in the blender. Scoop the flesh out of the avocado, and
put that in the blender too, with the dates, lemon juice, miso, and water.
Blend to a cream—add more water if you need to. Spoon the sauce over
the cucumber mixture and give it a good stir. Serve immediately.

*Serving suggestion: serve with curried parsnips. This cooling
cucumber and mint dish complements the heat of the curry.*

ARUGULA AND HIJIKI

Food processor • 10 minutes (1 hour soaking) • Serves 4

It may not be as fashionable as it once was, but you can't beat a plate of fresh arugula. With green leaves more than anything else, it pays to get them fresh out of the ground. Salads that are sold bagged in supermarkets are likely to have been washed in chlorine and sprayed with chemicals to preserve them, even if they're certified organic (see the brilliant book Not on the Label *by Felicity Lawrence if you're interested in finding out more on this). If you have the time and inclination, arugula is really easy to grow yourself, and only takes about three months.*

7 oz/200 g arugula

2 oz/60 g dried tomatoes (see page 171)

300 g/10 oz cauliflower pieces

4 oz/120 g pickled onions

1 oz/30 g hijiki, soaked 1 hour

2 tbsp olive oil

1 tbsp balsamic vinegar

1 tsp tamari

1 tsp agave syrup

Wash the arugula, and using scissors, snip the leaves into bite-sized lengths and put them in the salad bowl. Add in your dried tomatoes. If you're using shop-bought ones, rather than homemade, soak them in water for 20–60 minutes first. Process the cauliflower in the food processor until it is in tiny granular pieces—I call this cauliflower snow, and often sneak it into salads so that the children won't notice they're eating cauliflower. Add it into the salad bowl with the onions (any small pickled onion will do), the drained hijiki, and the dressing ingredients. Toss and serve immediately, before the arugula starts to wilt.

Serving suggestion: this makes a great dinner party dish, served with red pepper ketchup and broccoli and cucumber crudités, for a substantial gourmet dinner in under half an hour.

BROCCOLI BLISS

Food processor

10 minutes

Serves 4

This has all my favorite things in it!

4 small or 2 large broccoli heads

10 oz/300 g cauliflower

2 oz/60 g broccoli bits (see page 166)

1 oz/30 g dried sea vegetables

2 tbsp nutritional yeast flakes

1 tbsp Seagreens

2 tbsp tahini

2 tbsp flax oil

1 lemon, juiced

1 tbsp apple cider vinegar

Prepare the broccoli and cauliflower by chopping them coarsely, so they are in pieces about the same size as rice grains. Transfer to a serving bowl. Add in the broccoli bits, sea vegetables, nutritional yeast flakes, and Seagreens. In a small bowl, whisk up the tahini, flax oil, lemon juice, and apple cider vinegar. When you have a nice creamy dressing, pour it over the salad and stir it in thoroughly. Serve within a couple of hours.

Broccoli is such a staple in our house, we snack on it with dips,
put it in our salads, make pâté with it, stir it into soups,
juice it, even coat it in raw chocolate and eat it—choccoli!

EGG SALAD

Blender

10 minutes

Serves 2

*When I was in school, one of my friends used to have egg salad
sandwiches for lunch, and sometimes she would share them with me.
And for some reason this dish reminds me of Katharine Vaziri's egg
salad. You can spread it on Essene (sprouted) bread or crackers, but it's
so good I eat it as it is.*

10 oz/300 g cauliflower (about half a cauliflower)

1 large avocado

1 tbsp olive oil

1 clove garlic

2 tsp white miso

1 lemon, juiced

You want the cauliflower the size of rice grains; you can chop it up in the
food processor, the Vita-Mix, or by hand. Transfer it to a mixing bowl.
Remove the flesh from the avocado, and add it with all the remaining
ingredients to the blender, to blend to a cream. Make sure there are no
lumps of garlic in it; add water if you need to. Then transfer it to the bowl
with the cauliflower and give it all a good stir. Serve the same day.

Variation: you can substitute broccoli for some or all
of the cauliflower.

NOODLES

Spiral slicer • 20 minutes • Serves 4

These are amazingly authentic, like chow mein. They are also very satisfying, so you don't need to eat too many. Why is it everyone knows you can eat raw carrots, but people don't think of eating the other root vegetables raw? Squash is a good vegetable to add to your raw repertoire.

2 tbsp arame

1 medium-sized butternut squash

2 tbsp sesame seeds

2 tbsp poppy seeds

4 tbsp olive oil

1 tbsp tamari

4 oz/120 g sweet-corn kernels

16 cherry tomatoes, halved

Soak the arame in filtered water for 10–15 minutes while you prepare the squash. Top and tail it, then slice it into half, the round bulbous end and the narrower neck. Slice the neck lengthways into quarters. Slice the round end in half and scoop out the seeds, then slice it in half again. You should now have eight pieces of squash. Using a spiral slicer on the noodle section, process each piece and transfer to a mixing bowl. Because of the unusual shape of the vegetable, you are likely to have odd ends left over. Save these for another use: biscuits or soup. If you don't have a spiral slicer (or you are in a hurry), simply grate the squash. Add the remaining ingredients into the mixing bowl, along with the drained arame, and toss. You can serve as it is, or this also works well in pasta sauce (see page 148)

Squash is a member of the Cucurbit family, which includes cucumber, marrow, melon, pumpkin, gherkin, and loofah.

THAI RED CURRY

Blender, food processor • 20 minutes • Serves 2

Fresh coconut makes this rich and creamy and very warming with all those spices. Thai spices are easier to find now; supermarkets often stock a selection. If you can't get fresh coconut, you can substitute creamed coconut or coconut milk, but neither of these is raw.

2 tbsp arame

4 red peppers

2 carrots

2 tomatoes

1 stick celery

1 stick lemongrass

Small bunch cilantro

1 lime

4 oz/120 g fresh coconut pieces

4 fresh dates, pitted

2 cloves garlic

1 inch galangal

8 cups mushrooms

8 baby corn

1 1/2 oz/45 g mung bean or lentil sprouts

Prepare the arame by soaking it for 10–15 minutes. Remove the stem and seeds from the red pepper—chop into eighths. Top and tail the carrots, and chop into chunks. Quarter the tomatoes. Chop the celery into chunks. Chop the lemongrass and cilantro; juice the lime. Put the peppers, carrots, tomatoes, celery, lemongrass, cilantro, lime juice, coconut, dates, garlic, and galangal in the blender. The liquid from the vegetables should be plenty to make a thick sauce. Fine slice the mushrooms and baby corn, and transfer them to a mixing bowl with the bean sprouts, and the drained arame. Pour the red sauce over, and give it a good mix, making sure it's evenly stirred. Serve garnished with a sprig of fresh cilantro for a meal fit for the King of Thailand himself.

Baby corn is mainly grown in Thailand, and is cultivated by harvesting standard corn plants early, before they are mature.

SWEETHEART SALAD

Food processor

10 minutes

Serves 4

Happiness in a salad! The bright colors and sweet flavors of this dish are guaranteed to put a smile in your belly, especially in autumn when the nights are starting to draw in and raw food is maybe seeming a little more challenging.

1 apple

1 beetroot

4 carrots

$\frac{1}{2}$ sweet potato

2 tbsp macadamia nuts

4 oz/120 g sweet-corn kernels

4 tbsp mirin

2 tbsp sesame oil

1 tbsp Chinese 5 spice

Prepare your fruit and vegetables: remove the core of the apple, peel the beetroot, top and tail the carrots, and cut the sweet potato into chunks. Chop all into the size of rice granules. You can do this in a food processor with the S-blade, in a Vita-Mix, or by hand. Stir in the remaining ingredients. Eat right away, or marinate for a few hours first.

Macadamias are native to Australia and are generally pricey. But they are one of the tastiest, creamiest nuts around, with an unusual flavor and satisfying crunch.

KOHL RABI COLESLAW

Food processor

15 minutes

Serves 4

Kohl rabi, also known as turnip cabbage, is a white bulbous root vegetable with a sweet crunch that makes it a great candidate for coleslaw. Usually white, you can also sometimes find pretty purple ones too.

2 oz/60 g sea spaghetti

2 kohl rabi, grated

2 large carrots

1 onion

1 small cauliflower

1 avocado

1 tbsp Seagreens

2 tbsp nutritional yeast flakes

1 tbsp apple cider vinegar

2 tbsp hemp oil

Rinse the sea spaghetti, and soak in water for a few minutes to remove any excess salt. Top and tail the kohl rabi and carrots. Peel and quarter the onion. Grate the kohl rabi, carrots, and onion, and transfer to a mixing bowl. To prepare the cauliflower, take the heads and process them in a food processor with the S-blade until it's ground up into tiny pieces like snowflakes—we call this "cauliflower snow," a great addition to any salad and a good way to include cauliflower in your food if you're not keen on eating it in big chunks. Add the cauliflower to the mixing bowl. Cube the avocado flesh, and add that to the bowl. Sprinkle on your Seagreens, yeast flakes, vinegar, and hemp oil and give it all a good mix up. The coleslaw can be eaten right away or left to marinate for a few hours.

Michigan claims to be the kohl rabi capital of the world, and even holds kohl rabi festivals!

MY FAVORITE THINGS

No equipment needed

5 minutes

Serves 1

*Just a few of. . . . This is the perfect light lunch
for the woman on the run.*

1 oz/30 g dulse

1 oz/30 g alfalfa

10 pitted olives

2 oz/60 g arugula

1 tbsp hemp oil

1 tsp Liquid Aminos

1 tsp agave

1 tsp lemon juice

Rinse the dulse. Toss everything together in a bowl. Delicious served with rye bread (see page 158) spread with pumpkin seed butter.

*Alfalfa when fully grown is similar to hay, and is the third
most widely grown crop in the United States. Its primary
use is as animal feed for cattle, sheep, and horses.*

SAVORY ENTRÉES

Most of these recipes call for a dehydrator. If you feel sure you're going to be experimenting with raw foods for more than a few months, it's worth getting one of these "raw ovens." You'll have loads of fun making burgers, wraps, loaves, and cakes for you and your family. If you haven't got a dehydrator there are a few options available to you.

- You can lightly fry vegetable burgers in coconut oil (the only cold-pressed oil that is heat stable and so most suitable for frying). Just a few minutes on each side will warm them up and help them stick together without cooking them.

- You can place food under a low grill for a few minutes on each side. Again, make sure the food is lightly toasted on both sides without being cooked through.

- You can put the food in an airing cupboard or on top of a hot radiator for a day. This will dry it out a little.

- If it's hot out, you can try sun drying. Leave the food out in the sun for a day, but make sure the flies don't get on it, and bring it in if it starts to rain!

- Raw fooders often advise using the oven on the lowest heat with the door open. Just be careful not to leave it unattended, and make sure the oven doesn't get too hot.

However you choose to prepare them, the dishes in this section make a substantial addition to any meal and a welcome alternative to simple salads.

SPICY ALMOND BURGERS

Blender, dehydrator • 20 minutes (8–12 hours soaking,
12 hours drying) • Makes 12 burgers

*Flaxseeds are probably the best way of binding foods together in raw
food cuisine. A tablespoon or two of ground seeds is the surest way to
help your mixture stick together when you're making burgers, loaves,
pastries, biscuits, anything that needs a bit of firming up.*

2 tbsp ground flaxseeds

2 carrots

3 tomatoes

2 sticks celery

1 onion

2 red chilies

8 oz/250 g almonds, soaked 8–12 hours

1 tbsp tamari

Grind the flaxseeds in a coffee grinder or high-powered blender. Roughly
chop the carrots, tomatoes, celery, and onion so they fit in your blender.
After removing the seeds and stems, add the chilies to the blender, as well
as the almonds and tamari. Turn the blender on and puree until you have
no odd lumps of vegetable or nut left. Then add the flaxseeds and blend
again. Shape into patties with your hands, not more than 1 inch thick and
about 4 inches in diameter. It should make about twelve burgers. Put them
on the drying trays, and dry for 12 hours, until crunchy on both sides, but
tender in the middle.

*Flaxseeds also provide the easiest way to make raw
crackers. Simply soak your seeds in water, and when
they've absorbed as much as they are able (usually about
three times as much, weight for weight), then add your
favorite flavorings, sweet or savory, spread thinly
onto dehydrator sheets, and dry until crispy.*

BEETROOT BURGERS

Blender, dehydrator • 20 minutes (8–12 hours soaking,
6 hours dehydrating) • Serves 4; makes about 16 burgers

*Even people who don't like beetroot love these. The dehydrating process
brings out the natural sweetness of this wondrous vegetable.*

2 tbsp ground flaxseeds

4 beetroot

1 large carrot

1 tomato

1 red chili

$\frac{1}{2}$ onion

4 fresh dates, pitted

5 oz/150 g almonds, soaked 8–12 hours

1 tbsp tamari

4 fl oz/125 ml water

Grind the flaxseeds in a coffee grinder or high-powered blender. Top, tail, and peel the beetroot, and chop into chunks. Top and tail the carrot, and chop that into bite-sized chunks too. Cut the tomato into quarters. Remove the stem and seeds from the chili. If you have a high-powered blender, it will work best; otherwise, you're better off sticking to your food processor. Put in all the ingredients except the flaxseeds. You won't exactly get a puree, more of a mush. When you're confident there are no lumps of vegetable left in (you may get the odd stubborn bit of carrot or beetroot, just remove it), add the flaxseeds, which will bind the mixture. Shape into patties about 1 inch high and 4 inches wide. They should fill two drying trays. Dry for 4 hours, flip over, and dry for a further 2 hours. Eat within 24 hours. These are lovely burgers, moist and substantial. Serve with ketchup (red pepper or carrot, see pages 65–66) or a raw mayonnaise as a dip, and a side salad.

*Flaxseed tea is beneficial for the colon, strengthening
and cleansing. Soak 1 tablespoon of seeds in a pint of water,
simmer for 10 minutes, strain, and drink. Add lemon juice
and raw honey if you want to improve the taste.*

SUNNY BURGERS

Blender, dehydrator

15 minutes (4–8 hours soaking, 12 hours drying)

Makes 18 burgers

From the beautiful sunflower plant, sunflower seeds are probably the most popular seed to snack on. They're a great source of vitamin E, essential fatty acids, magnesium, and selenium.

8 oz/250 g sunflower seeds, soaked 4–8 hours

2 tbsp ground flaxseeds

2 sticks celery

1 onion

3 tomatoes

1 red chili

3 carrots, chopped

1 tbsp tamari

Soak sunflower seeds in advance. Grind flax in a coffee grinder or high-powered blender. Chop the celery, onion, and tomatoes. Remove the stem and seeds from the chili pepper. Put everything except the flaxseeds in the blender. Blend to a thick puree, and then add the flaxseeds in to stiffen the mixture. Using a tablespoon, spoon dollops of the mixture onto the dehydrator tray, and flatten down to about 1 inch fat and 4 inches in diameter. Arrange on a drying tray and dry for 8 hours. Flip and dry for another 4 hours.

I am often asked if flaxseeds on their own are sufficient to fulfill your EFA requirements. Two tablespoons of flax contain well over the RDA, but unless we have an extremely efficient digestive system, the body finds it hard to extract the necessary substances from the seeds, so I always advise supplementing with oils.

Love Burgers

Blender, dehydrator

15 minutes (8–12 hours soaking, 12 hours dehydrating)

Makes 12 burgers

These are beautifully sweet and creamy, and a wonderful romantic pink.
Serve them on Valentine's Day, or for a special lover's meal.

8 oz/250 g cashews, soaked 8–12 hours

2 red peppers

1 small cauliflower

$\frac{1}{2}$ onion

2 tsp white miso

Soak the cashews in advance. Prepare the peppers: remove the stem and seeds and chop into large chunks. Remove the leaves from the cauliflower and chop the florets into chunks. Put everything in the blender and blend to a thick cream. You shouldn't need to add water, as the peppers will turn to liquid. Take heaped tablespoons of the mixture and, using your hands, mold them into love heart shapes on the drying tray—about 1 inch high and 4 inches in diameter. Place on a drying tray and dehydrate for 12 hours, turning about two-thirds of the way through. Serve with red pepper ketchup (see page 65) drizzled around the plate to complete the effect.

We prefer white miso, or shiro miso, because it is less
salty and has a gentler flavor. But experiment with the
other types of miso, like mugi and hatcho. Natto miso
is a chutney that makes a delicious accompaniment
to salads or can be used in dressings.

HEMP BURGERS

Blender, dehydrator

15 minutes (4–8 hours soaking, 18 hours drying)

Makes 12 burgers

*Hemp seeds lend a distinctive depth to any dish. They are one of
the best sources of the essential fats omega-3 and omega-6,
as well as the hard-to-find gamma-linoleic acid.*

4 oz/120 g sprouted sunflower seeds (see Sprouting, page 49)

4 oz/120 g hemp seeds, soaked 4–8 hours

4 tomatoes

1 red pepper

Small bunch parsley

1 onion

1 tbsp garam masala

Sprout your sunflower seeds a day or two in advance. Presoak your hemp
seeds. Prepare your vegetables for the blender: remove any unwanted
stems, stalks, and seeds, and chop into large chunks. Put all the ingredients
in and blend to a thick pink cream. Spoon it out onto drying trays, making
patties, about 1 inch fat and 4 inches wide. Dry for 12 hours, then flip
them over and dry for another 6 hours.

*Hemp is not only a fantastic food, it's brilliant to put on
the skin too, healing, strengthening, and rejuvenating.*

LENTIL BURGERS

Blender, dehydrator

15 minutes (4–8 hours soaking, 12 hours drying)

Makes 12 burgers

Sprouted lentils are a great source of protein, and help to stabilize
blood sugar levels. They are rich in B vitamins and hard-to-find trace
minerals like molybdenum and manganese. We usually use green lentils,
but you can use the small black Puy lentils too. Red lentils will
not sprout as they have been cracked.

7 oz/200 g sprouted lentils (see Sprouting, page 49)

4 oz/120 g sunflower seeds, soaked 4–8 hours

2 oz/60 g ground flaxseeds

1 onion

Small bunch parsley

Small bunch basil

4 tbsp olive oil

1 tbsp miso

4 tbsp water

Sprout your lentils two or three days in advance. Presoak your sunflower seeds. Grind your flaxseeds in a coffee grinder or high-powered blender. Prepare the onion, parsley, and basil by chopping them loosely, and put them in the blender. Put everything else in the blender apart from the flaxseeds and process to thick batter. You may need to add a little more water. Add the flaxseeds in and blend again until the mixture has thickened. Shape into patties with your hands. With a spoon, shape into burgers about 1 inch high and 4 inches wide on your drying trays. Dry for 12 hours.

Onions and garlic are avoided by many yogis and Buddhists
because they are said to be overstimulating, or "rajasic" in
the Ayurvedic system, and not conducive to meditation.

TEMPURA

Blender, dehydrator • 30 minutes (4–8 hours soaking,
12 hours dehydrating) • Serves 4

*I used to adore tempura; it was one of my favorite treats. An Asian dish,
it is made by coating fresh vegetables in batter and deep-frying them.
One time we visited a Thai restaurant with the family, and I was
determined to recreate some raw tempura at home. After a bit of
trial and error, this is what I came up with. Serve warm, straight from
the dehydrator, with some Asian dipping sauce (see page 67).*

2 oz/60 g sunflower seeds, soaked 4–8 hours

2 oz/60 g pumpkin seeds, soaked 4–8 hours

4 red peppers

4 portobello mushrooms

2 oz/60 g flaxseeds

1 red chili, stem and seeds removed

2 cloves garlic

2 fresh dates, pitted

1 tbsp tamari

16 fl oz/500 ml water

You can presoak your sunflower and pumpkin seeds in the same bowl
together. Remove the stem and seeds from the pepper. Slice lengthways
into strips about $\frac{1}{2}$ inch wide. Slice the mushrooms into similar-size
pieces. To make the batter, put all the ingredients except the peppers and
mushrooms in the blender and process for a few minutes, until the mixture
starts to thicken. It should be kind of elastic. Transfer the batter and the
mushrooms and peppers to a mixing bowl, and mix thoroughly so they are
completely coated. Spread the mix over three or four drying trays, making
sure it is thinly and evenly distributed. Dry for 12 hours.

*Tempura was originally introduced to Japan by the Portuguese
in the fifteenth century, and the name is said to derive from
the Portuguese word temporo, which means seasoning.*

SPINACH CAKES

Blender, dehydrator • 5 minutes (4–8 hours soaking,
18 hours drying) • Makes 18 patties

*Spinach is an amazing source of nutrients, full of cancer-beating
flavonoids and carotenoids, and vitamins and minerals. One cup
of spinach contains 200 percent of the RDA of vitamin K, which is
important to help maintain bone health. If you can track down
loose spinach rather than the cut and bagged leaves,
it is much tastier and more nutritious.*

3 oz/90 g sesame seeds, soaked 4–8 hours

8 oz/250 g spinach

1 tsp tamari

1 tsp kelp

$\frac{1}{2}$ onion

4 fl oz/125 ml water

This is one of those easy peasy recipes. Presoak your sesame seeds. Then just chuck everything in the blender, and whiz for a couple of minutes, until all the seeds are ground in. Then spoon dollops of the mixture onto drying trays, and dry for 12 hours. Turn and dry on the other side for a further 6 hours.

*These little patties are particularly good
served with date chutney (see page 71).*

CILANTRO WRAPS

Blender, dehydrator

5 minutes (4–8 hours soaking, 12 hours drying)

Makes 4 wraps

*This is one of those simple things you can make that transforms
a humble salad into something spectacular. Even if you've only got
a few lettuce leaves in the fridge and a jar of tahini in the cupboard,
wrap them in one of these and you'll have a feast.*

5 oz/150 g flaxseeds, soaked in
16 fl oz/500 ml water for 4–8 hours

$\frac{1}{2}$ onion

Small bunch cilantro

1 tbsp cumin powder

1 tbsp garam masala

Soak the flaxseeds in the water; they will absorb it all and become gelatinous. If you haven't got 4 hours, even 20 minutes will do—you'll still need to add the full 16 fl oz (500 ml) of water to your mixture. Once they're ready, pop them in the blender with all the other ingredients. Blend to a puree, until there are no seeds discernable in the mix. Take a quarter of the mixture, and spread it in a round on a drying tray. Your round will nearly fill the tray—about 12 inches diameter. Make three more rounds, and dry for 8 hours. Flip over, and dry for another 4 hours. Don't let them go crispy—you want them to be nice and pliable, so you can fold them over. If you notice them starting to go crispy round the edge, take them out right away. Slide each round onto a plate. Spread with a dip, pâté, or some nut butter. Heap your favorite salad on top in a semicircle, so only one side is covered. Then fold the wrap in half across the middle, and eat like pita bread. Very satisfying! These will keep for a couple of days if need be.

*You can just cram your wrap with lettuce, olives,
and alfalfa, or try arugula and hijiki (page 121)
or broccoli bliss (page 122).*

BEAN CAKES

Blender, dehydrator

10 minutes (4–8 hours soaking, 18 hours dehydrating)

Makes 24 patties

These go great with date or cilantro chutney (see pages 70–71).
You can use a mix of lentils, aduki, mung beans, sunflower seeds,
or chickpeas in this recipe. If you haven't been organized enough
to sprout your own, one of the ready-made bags of mixed
sprouts available in whole foods stores is perfect.

8 oz/250 g mixed bean sprouts
(see Sprouting, page 49)

3 oz/90 g sesame seeds, soaked 4–8 hours

Small bunch cilantro

1 onion

2 tbsp olive oil

1 tbsp cumin powder

1 tbsp garam masala

1 tbsp tamari

Sprout your beans in advance. Presoak your sesame seeds. Prepare the cilantro and onion for the blender. Put all the ingredients in and blend to a thick puree. Add a little water if it won't blend, but keep it as thick as possible. Spoon dollops of the mixture onto a drying tray—about a tablespoon at a time. Ideally, they want to be about $\frac{1}{2}$ to 1 inch high—any fatter and they won't dry out. Dry for 12 hours, turn and dry for 6 hours more. The patties will stay fresh stored in an airtight container in the fridge for up to one week.

Coriander is the only plant to be classified as an herb and
a spice! The leaves (cilantro) are referred to as an herb,
while the seeds are used as a spice.

LENTIL AND SAGE SAUSAGES

Blender, dehydrator

10 minutes (18 hours drying)

Makes 12 sausages

This dish is very traditional!
It's great for lunches and picnics.

3 oz/90 g sprouted lentils (see Sprouting, page 49)

1 onion

Small bunch sage

4 tbsp olive oil

2 oz/60 g sesame seeds, soaked 4–8 hours

1 oz/30 g dried tomatoes (see page 171)

1 tbsp miso

Sprout your lentils two or three days in advance. Peel, top, and tail the onion and quarter it ready for the blender. Chop the sage loosely, and put everything in the blender. When you have a thick puree, take out about 1 tablespoon at a time and form into fat sausages on the trays, about 1 inch in diameter and 4 inches long. Place on drying trays and dry for 12 hours. Turn and dry for a further 6 hours. Serve with ketchup (red pepper or carrot, see pages 65–66).

The Latin name for sage is Salvia officinalis, which is derived
from salvere, the Latin for "to be saved," because of its
reputation as a medicinal plant.

CHICKPEA LOAF

Blender, dehydrator

10 minutes (4–8 hours soaking, 12 hours drying)

Serves 4

Sprouted chickpeas are a very calming, soothing, and reassuring food when blended into loaves, hummus, or soups. Just be careful when sprouting to keep the tails small: you want to have the bean bigger than the tail or you'll get a not-so-pleasant, woody flavor. Keep a little tail and you'll barely be able to tell the difference between a raw hummus and a cooked one.

5 oz/150 g sprouted chickpeas (see Sprouting, page 49)

3 oz/90 g sesame seeds, soaked 4–8 hours

2 carrots

1 onion

4 tbsp olive oil

1 small bunch parsley, finely chopped

2 tsp miso

8 tbsp water

Pasta sauce (see page 150) (optional)

Sprout your chickpeas two or three days in advance. Presoak your sesame seeds. Top and tail the carrots and onion, and prepare them for the blender. Put all the ingredients in the blender, and blend to a thick puree. Spoon out onto a drying tray, and shape into a loaf about $1\frac{1}{2}$ inches high, 6 inches wide, and 8 inches long. If you have the time and the inclination, make a serving of pasta sauce and spread it over the top. Dehydrate for 12 hours. Otherwise, you can make the sauce when you are ready to serve it, and spoon it over like gravy. Or serve with red pepper ketchup (see page 65).

Chickpeas are one of the top sources of dietary fiber. This dish contains virtually 100 percent of the daily requirement.

Mediterranean Stuffed Tomatoes

Food processor • 15 minutes • Serves 4

These are fun and easy to do, and make a great centerpiece for a summer lunch. Once again, it's the fresh herbs that add an extra dimension to this recipe and really make it a meal to savor. It goes well with sweetheart salad (page 126).

4 oz/120 g sprouted sunflower seeds (see Sprouting, page 49)

4 large beefsteak tomatoes

1 carrot

1 stick celery

1 bunch basil

1 bunch oregano

2 cloves garlic

1 tsp miso

1 lemon, juiced

2 tbsp olive oil

2 tbsp alfalfa sprouts (see Sprouting, page 49)

Sprout your sunflower seeds for two or three days. Slice the tops off the tomatoes and set aside (you don't need the lids). Using a paring knife carefully cut out the centers of the tomatoes, leaving a $\frac{1}{2}$ inch rim of flesh round the edge. Scoop out all the soft seedy innards with a spoon. You only need half of this pulp for the recipe; the rest you can save for a soup or sauce. Prepare the carrot, celery, basil, and oregano by chopping them into chunks to fit into your food processor. Pop them in, along with the sunflower sprouts, pulp of two tomatoes, garlic, miso, lemon juice, and olive oil. Process them so they still have a granular texture, and the ingredients are not completely blended up. Spoon this mixture into the four tomatoes. Garnish with alfalfa sprouts and serve immediately.

If you can't get fresh herbs, a dried Mediterranean blend of oregano, basil, rosemary, and thyme is delicious in a different way!

SPINACH AND MUSHROOM QUICHE

Food processor, blender • 40 minutes (8–12 hours soaking,
2 hours setting) • Serves 8

Raw pies and quiches are so much easier to make than cooked ones.
I often demonstrate them at workshops and people are amazed at how
quickly you can throw together such a tasty and impressive dish.
No rolling out pastry, no pre-baking, no boiling sauces,
no worrying about lumps or burnt crusts. Phew!

8 oz/250 g almonds

8 oz/250 g rolled oats

1 tbsp tahini

1 tbsp miso

1 tsp chili powder

1 tsp cumin powder

1 tbsp water

8 mushrooms (4 oz/120 g)

8 oz/250 g spinach

1 carrot

$\frac{1}{4}$ onion

$\frac{1}{2}$ avocado

1 tsp tamari

2 tbsp olive oil

4 fl oz/125 ml water

1 tbsp psyllium

First, make the crust: Put the almonds and oats in a food processor and
process as fully as possible. Add the tahini, miso, chili, and cumin, and
process again. If the mixture isn't sticking together, add a little water;
a tablespoon should be sufficient. When it's formed into a sticky dough,
press it into a large flan tin, lining the sides and base. Next, finely slice the
mushrooms and arrange them evenly in the pastry case.

To make the spinach cream, prepare the spinach, carrot, onion, and avocado, and put them in the blender. Add the tamari, olive oil, and water and blend. Once you have a thick cream, add the psyllium and blend again. The mixture will start to thicken. Pour it over the mushrooms, filling the almond pastry case. Pop it in the fridge for a couple of hours to allow the psyllium to set. Serve with a green salad like arugula and hijiki (see page 121).

Cumin seeds are quite different from the powder.
The seeds taste similar to fennel and dill, and are a super
addition to salads and soups. The powder, on the other hand,
is one of the predominant notes in curry powder and
has a warming, uplifting aroma and taste.

TOMATO QUICHE

Food processor, blender

30 minutes

Serves 8

Try this quiche with a green salad like simple salad (see page 108).

10 oz/300 g almonds

5 oz/150 g rolled oats

1 tbsp tahini

1 tbsp miso

2–4 tbsp water

8 mushrooms (8 oz/250 g)

3 oz/90 g olives

1 ear of corn

5 tomatoes

1 carrot

1 stick celery

$\frac{1}{4}$ cup dried tomatoes (see page 121)

2 dates

$\frac{1}{4}$ onion

1 tsp tamari

1 tbsp olive oil

1 tbsp apple cider vinegar

1 bunch basil

1 tbsp psyllium

Grind the almonds and oats in a high-powered blender or coffee grinder. Transfer to a mixing bowl and add tahini, miso, and water. Knead with your hands until you have firm dough. Press this into a large flan tin, lining the base and sides with a crust about $\frac{1}{4}$ inch thick. Next prepare your filling. Slice the mushrooms into pieces about $\frac{1}{4}$ inch thick. Arrange the pieces over your flan base. Sprinkle in the olives. Strip the corn kernels off the cob with a knife, and sprinkle those over the mushrooms and olives. The final step is to make the tomato sauce: Prepare your tomatoes, carrot, and celery for the blender, and blend up with the dried tomatoes, dates, onion, tamari, olive oil, vinegar, and basil. Blend to a smooth puree. Add the psyllium and blend again. The psyllium will start to set pretty quickly, so pour it over the flan base immediately. Leave for an hour or two in the fridge to set. The quiche will keep for three or four days in the fridge.

A French name for tomato is pomme d'amour, or apple of love, because they attribute aphrodisiacal qualities to the fruit.

CASHEW PANCAKES

Blender, dehydrator
15 minutes (8–12 hours soaking, 8–10 hours dehydrating)
Makes 8 pancakes

*This is based on a recipe shared by a raw mum from England named
Karen Rodgers. They're amazingly authentic—spread with agave
syrup and white almond butter for a Shrove Tuesday treat.
The temptation is to eat heaps of them, but it's probably wise
to stick to two per person as they're very rich.*

8 oz/250 g cashews, soaked 8–12 hours
16 fl oz/500 ml water
2 tsp vanilla extract
1 tsp tamari
4 fresh dates, pitted
1 tbsp psyllium powder

Presoak your cashews. Put everything except the psyllium in the blender
and blend to a runny cream. Keep your blender on for a few minutes to
ensure the mix is really smooth, not bitty. When it's ready, add the psyllium
and blend again briefly. Spoon out onto drying trays immediately, before
the psyllium starts to set. You can fit two pancakes to a tray, about 6 inches
in diameter. Spread it fairly thin, and it should make eight pancakes. Dry
for 6 hours, then flip over and dry for another 2–4 hours on the other side.
Serve warm, straight out of the dehydrator. Leftovers (ha!) will keep for a
day or two in the fridge.

*The cashew is the seed of the cashew apple fruit.
Not commonly eaten in the United States or Europe, the
fruit is very popular in Brazil and the Caribbean.*

CHILI

Blender

20 minutes

Serves 2

You can serve this in two ways: Add some ready-prepared vegetables, like sliced mushrooms, cubed peppers, broccoli florets, sweet-corn kernels, or shredded spinach leaves, and stir them in to make a vegetable chili. Or leave it as is and serve tacos. Get some romaine lettuce leaves as your taco shells. Fill each leaf with the chili, and top with a raw mayonnaise (try cashew cream cheese, page 75) and some alfalfa sprouts.

1 large or 2 small beetroot

3 tomatoes

1 red chili pepper, stem and seeds removed

4 fresh dates, pitted

1 tbsp apple cider vinegar

2 tbsp olive oil

1 tsp tamari

$\frac{1}{4}$ onion

2 cloves garlic

2 tbsp dulse flakes

1 oz/30 g mixed bean sprouts (see Sprouting, page 49)

Top, tail, and peel the beetroot. If you have a high-powered blender, you can just cube it at this stage in preparation; otherwise, grate it and set it aside. Put the tomatoes, chili, dates, vinegar, olive oil, tamari, onion, and garlic in the blender, and blend to a puree. Once it's smooth, add the grated beetroot and dulse flakes and stir in by hand. If you're using the blender, you can add the cubed beetroot and dulse, and blend it on a medium setting—this creates a sort of minced-beef effect, where the beetroot is half blended, half chunky. Add the bean sprouts, and stir in by hand.

Chili peppers are thought to have been cultivated in Central and South America for more than 7,000 years.

PASTA SAUCE

My favorite all-time recipe is pasta sauce. Now I know every raw chef has their own pasta sauce recipe, and you may think there can't be much to it, just chuck some tomatoes and basil in the blender, and there you have it. But believe me, there is something about this recipe that is unbeatable. No matter how many times I make it, I always end up scraping the bowl and licking the jug to get every last precious drop out. It was also one of the first recipes I ever developed. My three-year-old son was a very picky raw eater (note to other moms with the same problem: it was a phase, it passes, just stick with it). So I had to invent ways of hiding raw foods that he would find palatable in his dinner. One of his favorite dinners was wheat-free pasta (usually corn or rice), drowned in this sauce.

Obviously, the main ingredients are tomatoes—some fresh and some dried. You can either buy them sun-dried in packets, or dry them yourself in the dehydrator; I prefer to dry them myself because (a) then I know they're really raw, and relatively fresh, and (b) it's cheaper. Dried tomatoes add a real richness and depth of flavor to any sauce. Then I add carrot and celery, as a way of adding body to the sauce, and sneaking some extra vegetables into my children's bodies. They would refuse to eat celery in its natural state, but they get plenty this way, hidden in sauces, burgers, and the like. I also put in a handful of dulse, and a little kelp. We eat tons of sea vegetables, which are so important as a source of minerals, and are a wonderfully satisfying addition to savory dishes. Did you know dulse has fifteen times more calcium than cow's milk, weight for weight? Next in the blender are dates and onion. For some reason, this unlikely pair of ingredients really works together, creating a mouth-watering blend of sweet and spice. Finally, you want a little apple cider vinegar, a dash of tamari, and a drizzle of olive oil, to ensure a vibrant, tangy sauce.

We have it every week, because the variations are endless. If I'm serving it for the children, I would just leave it like that, and pour it over the pasta. Or sometimes they have "baked beans": sprouted chickpeas, which have been cooked in water for half an hour to soften them. But for my husband and I, I tweak it a little, and transform it into a whole new dish. For a basic pasta, I add a bunch of basil, half a red chili, and a clove of garlic per person. Pour it over chopped vegetables, and serve with a sprinkling of your favorite raw cheese substitute, or a handful of pine nuts. Try courgetti (courgettes, that is zucchini, done in the spiral slicer like spaghetti), or carrotelli (carrots done in the spiral slicer like tagliatelli). Butternut squash also makes great noodles when done in the spiral slicer. Another obvious one is to use it as a sauce on a pizza base. There are plenty of raw pizza base recipes around; you could try simply whizzing up tomatoes and flaxseeds, then shape the mix into thin rounds, and dehydrate. If you haven't got time to make bases, mix the usual pizza toppings into the sauce, sweet corn, mushrooms, and olives, say, and use to stuff peppers—pizza peppers! For a raw chili, add one whole red chili per person, and mix some finely grated beetroot and carrot into your sauce, along with a big handful of bean sprouts. Fancy a curry? Add one clove of garlic, an equal-sized piece of ginger, one red chili, and a teaspoon of curry powder. Mix in some vegetables—mushrooms, cauliflower, broccoli, and red pepper is a good combination. And finally, my favorite variation is Thai red curry (page 125): add in traditional Thai seasonings, such as galangal, lime, lemongrass, cilantro, and coconut.

By my count, that makes eleven different ways to use this sauce, and there are bound to be others that I have forgotten, and more that you can think of. If that hasn't tempted your taste buds and got you reaching for the blender, I don't know what will!

BASIC RECIPE FOR PASTA SAUCE

Blender

10 minutes

Serves 1

This is a perfect sauce for every occasion.

3 tomatoes

1 carrot

1 stick celery

1 tbsp dulse

$\frac{1}{2}$ avocado

2 tbsp dried tomatoes

$\frac{1}{2}$ tsp kelp

1 fresh date, pitted

$\frac{1}{4}$ onion

1 tsp apple cider vinegar

1 tsp tamari

1 tbsp olive oil

Roughly chop tomatoes, carrot, and celery. Rinse the dulse. Put everything in the blender and blend till smooth. That's it!

It is often asserted that the lycopene in tomatoes is only bioavailable when cooked. This is not strictly accurate. Although it is true to say raw tomatoes are not a good source of this valuable antioxidant, it can still be utilized if the tomatoes are juiced or dried (that is, sun-dried tomatoes).

PIZZA PEPPERS

Blender

15 minutes

Serves 4 as a main dish or 8 as a side dish

This dish is perfect if you don't have time to make pizza bases.

2 portions pasta sauce (see page 150)

4 red peppers

1 small head broccoli

3 oz/90 g spinach

2 oz/60 g corn

2 oz/60 g olives

2 oz/60 g pine nuts

Prepare the pasta sauce. Slice the peppers in half lengthways and remove all seeds and stems. Chop the broccoli into small bite-sized pieces, about the size of cashew nuts. Fine slice the spinach. In a mixing bowl, stir up the pasta sauce, broccoli, spinach, corn, olives, and pine nuts so everything is equally distributed. Spoon into the peppers. Serve immediately, or dehydrate for a few hours to warm through and bring out the flavors.

If you are making this for guests, use a mixture of yellow, red, and orange peppers to make it look even more attractive.

TRICOLOR PASTA

Spiral slicer, blender • 15 minutes • Serves 4

*This pasta is delicious immediately after it is prepared,
but it can also be eaten a day or two later when the vegetables
have softened and the flavors improved.*

2 portions pasta sauce (see page 150)

2 zucchini

3 carrots

1 beetroot

Prepare the pasta sauce. Top and tail the zucchini, carrots, and beetroot. Peel the beetroot. If you have a spiral slicer, you can make amazing noodles with your vegetables. If you don't own one of these handy gadgets, you can make noodles by just using a vegetable peeler: peel the vegetables downward in long strips to make tagliatelle-like strips. Or if you're in a hurry, just grate everything in a food processor. Whatever you use, you should have three piles of vegetables—green, red, and orange. Stir these into your sauce. This will keep for a few days in the fridge.

*The flowers from the zucchini plant are a delicacy that can be
eaten raw in salads, or deep-fried in batter like tempura.*

GOURMET PASTA

Spiral slicer, food processor • 20 minutes • Serves 2

This is a gorgeous, "meaty" pasta.

2 portions pasta sauce (see page 150)

1 carrot

1 zucchini

3 oz/90 g green leaf (for example, arugula)

1 avocado

7 oz/200 g oyster mushrooms

2 tbsp olives

2 oz/60 g dried tomatoes (see page 171)

2 tbsp alfalfa sprouts

2 oz/60 g cashew nuts

Prepare the pasta sauce. Using your spiral slicer, make vegetable ribbons with the carrot and zucchini. If you don't have a spiral slicer, you can use a potato peeler instead: Top and tail the vegetables, and peel away at the flesh repeatedly—these peelings are your ribbons or "pasta." Put the ribbons in a large mixing bowl. Next prepare your green leaf—if the leaves are big, you may want to trim it by just chopping it with scissors—and add it into the bowl. Cube the avocado flesh, and scoop it out into the bowl. Oyster mushrooms have a very strong flavor. Fine slice them, so they add a meaty texture to your dish without being overpowering. Add them to the mix, along with the olives, dried tomatoes, and pasta sauce. Give it all a good stir with a spoon, to get it evenly coated. Divide the mixture between two serving bowls. Chop the nuts in the food processor, so that they are not ground but are in pieces about the same size as grated cheese. Garnish each serving with a handful of alfalfa and a sprinkling of cashews.

In England, wild garlic can be found in the hedgerows in spring. It is a soft green leaf with a pungent garlic aroma, and you can eat the garlic-flavored flowers too. If you are visiting the British Isles, try using wild garlic leaves in your gourmet pasta!

BREAD AND CRACKERS

Unfortunately, there is no way round it, you really do need a dehydrator for the recipes in this section. There are cheap small ones on the market, which are good if you are just dabbling. However, if you think you are serious about raw foods, the only option is the Excalibur nine-tray food dehydrator. Nine trays may seem like a lot, but dehydrating usually involves bulk quantities, and you will be amazed at how quickly you can fill it up. They come in black and white and are about the size of a microwave oven. When they're on (usually for 12–24-hour periods) they emit a low humming sound, caused by the fan at the back of the machine. They also tend to fill the house with lovely home-baking smells—anything with cinnamon or onion in it is particularly pungent. I think they're set to be the latest trend. A few years ago, juicing was just for the health freaks, now every home has a juicer. In the same way, I think people are going to start cottoning on to what fun you can have with a dehydrator, and they'll soon become the latest must-have kitchen accessory.

It is perfectly possible to be raw without a dehydrator. I was raw for six years before I got one. Purists argue that dehydrated food shouldn't be classed as raw anyhow, and it's certainly true that you shouldn't eat too much of it. But if you want raw bread, crackers, or cookies, it really is indispensable.

CRUNCHY QUINOA CRACKERS

Blender and dehydrator

15 minutes (8–12 hours soaking, 18 hours dehydrating)

Makes about 30 crackers

Quinoa (pronounced keen-wah) is an ancient Aztec grain.
It is a complete protein, and one of the few grains that is not glutinous
in its cooked form. It is tricky to sprout, but if you get a good batch,
it is a lovely light addition to salads.

4 oz/120 g sprouted quinoa
(see Sprouting, page 49)

2 oz/60 g flaxseeds, soaked overnight
(see below)

1 tsp tamari

2 tbsp olive oil

2 tbsp nori flakes

Sprout the quinoa a couple of days in advance. Soak the flaxseeds overnight in 8 fl oz (250 ml) water. They will form a gloopy mass. Spoon it into the blender, along with the tamari and olive oil, and blend until you have a cream and you can't see any seeds left. Stir in the quinoa grains and nori flakes by hand. Spread onto two dehydrator trays and dry for 12 hours. Slice, turn, and dehydrate for a further 6 hours.

You can also eat quinoa leaves, which are similar to spinach
and chard as they are from the same family.

OATCAKES

Grinder, food processor, dehydrator

10 minutes (12 hours dehydrating)

Makes 12 oatcakes

Although oats are glutinous, like wheat, people are much less likely to have a problem digesting them than they are with wheat. If you buy raw oat groats and sprout them, then the starches turn to sugars and the gluten content becomes negligible. However, in this recipe they haven't been sprouted, so best not to eat too many. But they really capture that crumbly wholesome feel of traditional oatcakes; one or two spread with tahini or jam (see page 219) make a lovely snack.

5 oz/150 g ground oat groats

2 tbsp olive oil

$\frac{1}{4}$ tsp sea salt

4 fl oz/125 ml water

Grind your oats into flour using a coffee grinder or high-powered blender. Mix all the ingredients by hand or in a food processor. Using a teaspoon, spoon the mix onto a dehydrator tray, flattening out each spoonful into a round about 3 inches in diameter—best not to try it in sheets as it's very crumbly. Also, don't make them too thin or they will crumble when you try and turn them over. Dry for 10 hours, then flip them over with a spatula, and do them for a couple more hours on the other side.

Oats are a staple food in Scotland, whereas in England until relatively recently they were considered to be only good enough for animal feed. The English had a saying that went, "Oats are only fit to be fed to horses and Scotsmen"; the Scottish reply was, "And England has the finest horses, while Scotland has the finest men."

MISO BREAD

Juicer with blank plate, dehydrator

15 minutes (3 days sprouting, 4 hours soaking,
24 hours dehydrating)

Serves 8

*Essene bread (that is, sprouted bread) is one of the few things that
does work in an oven if you don't have access to a dehydrator.
Switch your oven to the lowest temperature, and leave the bread in
for 12–24 hours. It's heated too much to be considered
raw this way, but it's still great bread.*

6 oz/180 g sprouted wheat (see Sprouting, page 49)

2 tbsp pumpkin seeds

2 tbsp sunflower seeds

2 tbsp sesame seeds

2 tbsp hemp seeds

$\frac{1}{2}$ onion

1 tsp miso

Sprout the wheat three days in advance. You need a gear juicer (as opposed
to a centrifugal juicer) for this recipe, to really puree the ingredients. Soak
all the seeds for 2 to 4 hours, then rinse and drain. Push them through your
juicer with the blank plate on; they should go through easily because
they've been soaked. Then push the onion through, and then all the wheat.
Add the miso into the bowl, and mix in with your hands, kneading all the
ingredients together like dough, making sure the seeds are evenly mixed in.
On a dehydrator tray, shape into a loaf about $1\frac{1}{2}$ inches high and dry for 18
hours. Turn and dry for another 6 hours. Serve with soup or a salad (it goes
well with arugula).

*If you want to avoid wheat, even in its sprouted form,
you can substitute Kamut or spelt in this recipe,
which are ancient grains very similar to wheat.*

RYE BREAD

Juicer with blank plate, dehydrator
10 minutes (3 days sprouting, 18–24 hours dehydrating)
Makes 1 loaf

*Rye bread has a distinctive, interesting flavor. When grains are sprouted,
the starches are turned into sugars, so sprouted breads are suitable
for people who have gluten intolerance.*

11 oz/330 g sprouted rye grain
(see Sprouting, page 49)

4 tbsp olive oil

1 tbsp Seagreens

2 tbsp nutritional yeast flakes

1 tbsp tamari

Sprout the rye grain for three days. Using a heavy-duty juicer, push the
grain through with the blank plate on. Transfer to a mixing bowl, and add
the remaining ingredients, kneading with your hands until they are thoroughly mixed. On a dehydrator tray, shape the dough into a loaf about $\frac{1}{2}$
inch high. Dry for 12 hours, then flip over, and dry for a further 6–12
hours, until crusty. Serve spread with tahini and topped with alfalfa
sprouts. Lovely with a green salad like simple salad (page 108).

*Rye is one of the more recently cultivated grains, originating
as an agricultural crop in Germany around 2,000 years ago,
and today is mostly grown in Russia.*

LEBANESE CAULIFLOWER CRACKERS

Blender, dehydrator

15 minutes (8–12 hours presoaking, 18 hours dehydrating)

Makes about 40 crackers

These are deliciously light, wholesome crackers. Zaatar is a traditional Lebanese flavoring, which you can find in a specialty grocers. It is a blend of thyme, sumac, and sesame seeds.

5 oz/150 g Brazil nuts

2 oz/60 g flaxseeds

1 medium cauliflower

2 lemons

2 tbsp zaatar

Soak the Brazil nuts and flaxseeds overnight in 16 fl oz (500 ml) water. They will swell and absorb all the water. Roughly chop the cauliflower (you can use the leaves for juicing, they're very nutritious). Juice the lemons. Put the nuts, seeds, cauliflower, and lemon juice in the blender and blend to a thick cream. Stir in the zaatar by hand, making sure it's mixed right through to the bottom. You can actually eat it like this; I like the taste, and the flaxseeds are very beneficial when eaten this way. You could have some with a salad and eat it with a spoon. But if you're making crackers, spread the mix as thin as it will go on a dehydrator tray, in one big square. It should cover two trays. After about 12 hours, score through the big square into smaller squares; you should be able to get about 20 out of each tray. Dehydrate for about another 6 hours, until they're really crispy. These are so tasty and flavorsome, you can eat them on their own—they make good snacks.

You can make these crackers with other vegetables too. Try making zucchini crackers by substituting 1 pound (500 g) zucchini for the cauliflower, and omit the lemon juice.

OLIVE CRACKERS

Blender, dehydrator

5 minutes (3 days sprouting, 16–18 hours dehydrating)

Makes 30 crackers

These are gorgeous, rich, substantial, healthy—
the perfect between-meal snack, or accompaniment to salads.

11 oz/330 g sprouted rye
(see Sprouting, page 49)

2 oz/60 g ground flaxseed

7 oz/200 g pitted olives

$1/_2$ onion, peeled and chopped

Sprout your rye grain for three days. Grind your flaxseeds. Put everything in the blender and blend to a cream. Spread thin onto a couple of dehydrator trays and dry for 12 hours. Score into crackers, about 16 to each sheet, turn, and dry for another 4-6 hours. Store in an airtight container for up to two weeks.

Olives are one of the most ancient foods known; they play
an important role in Greek mythology and are
mentioned frequently in the Bible.

TRAFFIC LIGHT CRACKERS

Blender, dehydrator
30 minutes (8–12 hours presoaking, 18 hours dehydrating)
Makes about 40 crackers

*These crackers offer a great way to get more vegetables into children—
they love playing with the different color crackers and making
patterns on their plates. Just make sure they don't eat all
the red ones and leave all the spinach ones!*

5 oz/150 g Brazil nuts
2 oz/60 g flaxseeds
Add one of the following vegetables:
3 red peppers to make red biscuits
2 large carrots to make orange-yellow biscuits
8 oz/250 g spinach to make green biscuits

Presoak the Brazil nuts and flaxseeds in 16 fl oz (500 ml) water. Put the nuts, seeds, and whichever vegetable you are using in the blender (if you are not using a Vita-Mix you may want to grind the nuts and seeds first, for ease of blending). Add water if necessary. The red pepper mix shouldn't need any water, the carrot mix definitely will, and the spinach just a little.

Using a teaspoon, make small circles of the mix on the dehydrator tray—only about $1\frac{1}{4}$ inches in diameter, the right size for fitting 3 on a plate in a vertical row. If you want to make proper traffic lights, then you need to make three batches of biscuits—pepper for red, carrot for orange-yellow, and spinach for green.

Dehydrate for 12–18 hours until slightly crispy. Each batch makes at least 40 little crackers. They will keep for weeks in an airtight container.

*Brazil nuts are not farmed, but only grow wild in the Amazon
rainforest. Because the rainforests are being cut down, there
are actually fewer and fewer Brazil nuts available in the
global marketplace, while demand for this healthy food
increases, which is why the price of Brazils has
risen so much over the past decade.*

TOMATO CRACKERS

Blender, dehydrator

5 minutes (8–12 hours presoaking, 18 hours dehydrating)

Makes 20 crackers

This is a gorgeous, tangy cracker, bursting with flavor.

5 oz/150 g flaxseeds, soaked 8–12 hours
in 16 fl oz (500 ml) water

6 tomatoes, quartered

2 oz/60 g dried tomatoes (see page 171)

1 lemon, juiced

1 tbsp tamari

4 cloves garlic

$\frac{1}{2}$ oz/15 g dulse flakes

Presoak your flaxseeds. Pour all the ingredients, except the dulse flakes, in the blender and blend until the flaxseeds and tomato are amalgamated into a beautiful pink mixture. Stir in the dulse flakes by hand. Spread onto two drying trays, and dry for 12 hours. Score each sheet into 4 crackers by 5 crackers, and flip them over. Dry for a further 6 hours, until crisp. Stored in an airtight container, they will keep for up to a week.

*There are over a thousand varieties of tomato! They come
in a huge range of sizes and colors, including yellow,
orange, green, purple, and brown.*

SPELT AND CILANTRO CRACKERS

Blender, dehydrator

10 minutes (3 days sprouting, 18 hours dehydrating)

Makes 40 crackers

Spelt is an ancient form of wheat, popular with people who have wheat intolerance. It is very similar to wheat, with a delightful nutty flavor. These make a very tasty, wholesome snack.

8 oz/250 g sprouted spelt grain
(see Sprouting, page 49)

2 oz/60 g ground flaxseed

1 onion

Small bunch cilantro

2 tbsp olive oil

1 tbsp tamari

8 fl oz/250 ml water

Sprout the spelt for three days. Grind the flaxseed. Peel and chop the onion. Loosely chop the cilantro. Put everything together in the blender and blend to a thick puree. Spread onto two drying trays, fairly thin. Dry for 12 hours. Score each sheet into 5 squares by 4 squares, and flip them over. Dry for a further 6 hours. Store in an airtight container; they will keep for a couple of weeks.

Although cultivated for around 7,000 years, spelt fell out of favor probably because it is tougher than wheat and so harder to process. It has been made more popular in recent years as people look for wheat alternatives.

SAND CRACKERS

Blender, dehydrator

5 minutes (8–12 hours soaking, 12 hours dehydrating)

Makes about 30 crackers

My son named these, because they look like sand, and they
taste of the seaside too, with the kelp and sea vegetables.
And of course, you can put two together and make a sandwich!

5 oz/150 g Brazil nuts, soaked 8–12 hours

2 oz/60 g ground flaxseeds

1 tbsp miso

1 tsp kelp powder

16 fl oz/500 ml water

4 tbsp dried sea vegetables

Presoak your brazil nuts the day before. Put all the ingredients apart from the sea vegetables in a blender, and blend for a few minutes until it has thickened (you may need to add more water). Stir in the sea vegetables by hand, making sure they are evenly distributed throughout the mixture. Shape into flat cookies about 2 inches across and dehydrate for about 12 hours.

Brazil nuts are the richest natural source of selenium, a mineral
that is particularly important for men's health and has been
linked with the prevention of prostate cancer.

LISA'S RAW INDIAN BARS

Blender, dehydrator

5 minutes (8–12 hours soaking, 12 hours dehydrating)

Makes 30 bars

This is based on a recipe that my wonderful friend Lisa Gylsen sent to me.
The flavor is a bit strong for children, but very popular with adults.

7 oz/200 g cashews, soaked 8–12 hours

1 red onion

4 oz/120 g fresh coconut

1 clove garlic

2 lime leaves

1 tsp miso

1 tbsp curry powder

1 tsp cinnamon

4 lemons, juiced

Soak the cashews overnight. Peel and chop the onion. Chop the coconut into small pieces to make it easy for your blender to break down. Put everything in the blender and keep mashing until there are no lumps of coconut left or stray bits of lime leaf. Spread the mixture on drying trays and dehydrate for 12 hours. Score into rectangles about 4 inches long and 2 inches wide. Store in an airtight container in the fridge.

Lime leaves come from a wild lime tree and are also known as
kaffir lime leaves. They are usually sold dried or frozen.

EXTRAS

Here are more reasons to get a dehydrator. None of these recipes are essentials, but I keep them handy to liven up a salad, and add a bit of bite and crunch. They make good snacks too—just a handful or two will fill a gap between meals and provide a nourishing and sustaining burst of energy. They're quick and easy to make, and really worth trying. It's the little touches like these that can help you stay raw by adding a bit of variety and preventing you from getting into a rut with your food.

I haven't put in serving sizes for any of these recipes because it's impossible to say how much you'll get through: some people will want to make a batch and keep them in the cupboard for a month, using them sparingly as a salad garnish, others will sit down and eat the whole recipe in one or two sittings just as they are!

Broccoli Bits

Blender, dehydrator • 10 minutes (12 hours dehydrating)

Broccoli is one of my favorite foods. It's so full of nutrients, it's practically a super food in its own right. When I was breastfeeding Zachary, I couldn't get enough of it; I'd drink half a pint of broccoli juice every day. So I thought I'd try drying it and seeing what I came up with. Well, I hit the jackpot. These little nibbles are so tasty, and best of all the boys eat loads. If you have a child who is fussy about their greens, this is a marvellous way to get some of that tip-top nutrition in them.

4 lb/2 kg broccoli

1 onion, peeled and chopped

4 lemons, juiced

4 fl oz/125 ml olive oil

Put the broccoli, onion, lemon juice, and olive oil in the blender and blend to a puree. You can add more olive oil if you need to, or just if you want the broccoli bits to turn out richer. Spread on a dehydrator sheet and dry for 12 hours. When it's done, just break pieces off the tray; they'll crumble into chunks. Store them in an airtight container. You can snack on the broccoli bits as they are, like chips, or sprinkle them on salads. The lemon juice makes them wonderfully tangy.

The name broccoli comes from the Italian
and means "cabbage sprout"!

CARROT CRUNCH

Grater, dehydrator • 5 minutes (12 hours dehydrating)

We used to always have Bombay mix in the cupboard to add to our
salads for a bit of crunch. It was one of the last cooked foods to
go in our house. Now I have this instead.

1 lb/500 g carrots

3 tbsp olive oil

2 tbsp garam masala

2 tbsp poppy seeds

2 tbsp sesame seeds

Top and tail the carrots, and grate them finely. In a bowl, mix all the ingredients together so that the seeds coat the carrots. Be careful not to use too much oil or the carrots will not become crispy. Spread onto dehydrator trays (it should cover two trays), and dry for 12 hours. Store in an airtight container.

Carrots are recognized to be one of the best dietary sources
of vitamin A: 100 grams of carrots contains about six times
the RDA of this important vitamin.

CURRY CRUNCH

Dehydrator • 5 minutes (2 days sprouting, 12 hours dehydrating)

Like the previous recipe, this evolved as a replacement for Bombay mix.
It's so yummy, you can just eat a handful or two as a snack.

10 oz/300 g sprouted buckwheat (see Sprouting, page 49)
2 tbsp curry powder
2 tbsp sesame oil

Sprout the buckwheat for around two days so it has a little tail. In a bowl, mix it with the curry powder and sesame oil so the sprouts are evenly coated. Spread onto your dehydrator trays and dry for 12 hours. Stored in an airtight tub, these will keep for a good few weeks.

Dehydrated buckwheat makes great flour for raw pastries
and cakes: just sprout, dehydrate, and grind and use
instead of oats or nuts in any recipe.

NORI CHIPS

Blender, dehydrator • 5 minutes (18 hours dehydrating)

Tomato chips are a staple in our kitchen. But as tomatoes are
very acidic, I wasn't too happy about the boys having a lot of them.
So I developed this recipe instead. Cucumbers are very
alkaline and cleansing.

1 lb/500 g tomatoes
1 lb/500 g cucumbers
2 tbsp nori flakes

Blend the tomatoes and cucumbers together to a liquid. Then briefly whiz in the nori flakes so they're evenly distributed throughout the mixture.

Spread onto dehydrator trays (makes about four trays). Dry for 18 hours. Snap into pieces; how big you want them is up to you. Store in an airtight container and keep for up to a month.

You can make just cucumber chips by blending up cucumbers on their own, but they're not as tasty and the sheets turn out paper thin because cucumber is so watery.

SWEET POTATO CHIPS

Fine slicer, dehydrator • 5 minutes (12 hours dehydrating)

I've tried turning every vegetable you can think of into chips—beetroot, parsnip, carrot, and more. The trick is to slice them as thinly as possible; you need a machine with a really fine blade. But even then, most of them turn out woody and not that crispy—not great. The only two that work really well for me are sweet potato and zucchini. You can use any sort of spice you want on them.

1 large sweet potato

1 tbsp olive oil

1 tbsp curry powder

I usually don't bother peeling the sweet potato for this, just wash it. Slice it either with a mandolin or the fine blade on your food processor. Transfer it to a bowl, and mix in the oil and curry powder so the pieces of potato are evenly coated and none of them are sticking together. Don't use too much oil or they won't go crispy. Spread them evenly on your dehydrating trays— it doesn't matter if they overlap a bit, just as long as they're not all heaped on top of one another. Dry for 12 hours, then store in an airtight container. They only stay crispy for a day or two, which is why I haven't given a very large amount—you need to eat them all right away.

Never mind the fancy packs of fried root vegetable chips that cost a fortune—these are just as good and cost pennies!

ZUCCHINI CHIPS

Fine slicer, dehydrator • 5 minutes (12 hours dehydrating)

These are my favorites. Light and tasty,
we often have a handful each with tea.

1 lb/500 g zucchini

1 tbsp sesame oil

2 tbsp Chinese 5 spice

Top and tail the zucchini. Using a mandolin or the fine blade on your food processor, slice them up. Then transfer them to a mixing bowl and coat them evenly with the oil and spice. Spread on the dehydrator trays and dry for 12 hours. Store in an airtight container and eat within a day or two.

These are perfect with guacamole (see page 64)
or cilantro chutney (see page 70).

DULSE CHIPS

Dehydrator • 5 minutes (12 hours dehydrating)

You can hardly get more nutritious than dulse. These are surprisingly
tasty, and unlike their deep-fried alternative, no guilt involved.

1 packet dulse

1 tbsp olive oil

Rinse the dulse and separate the strands. Put it in a bowl and lightly coat with the olive oil. Spread onto drying trays and dry for 12 hours. You don't need any salt as sea vegetables are naturally salty. You can also try this with wakame, although it needs soaking for about 10 minutes first. These are best eaten right away, but you can probably get away with storing them in an airtight container for a few days.

Sea vegetables are not just an important part of Japanese cuisine. In fact, they are enjoyed by most countries with extensive coastal regions such as Ireland, Iceland, France, Australia, and Hawaii.

DRIED TOMATOES

Dehydrator • 10 minutes (24 hours dehydrating)

People were always asking me if it was possible to make sun-dried tomatoes in the dehydrator, and I could never figure out a way of doing it. If you slice them in a food processor, you lose a lot of the juice and seeds, and they come out too thin and chewy. If you cut them in half, like the shop-bought ones, they just take forever to do, and never fully dry out. It took me a long while to discover that you could just slice them thickly, and get that meaty effect you get in the sun-dried ones.

16 tomatoes

Cut each tomato into slices about $\frac{1}{2}$ inch thick. I usually find I get about four slices out of each tomato. You can use beef tomatoes and get more slices, or cherry tomatoes simply halved work well. Arrange them on a drying tray—you should get about 8 tomatoes to a tray. Dry for 24 hours—some fatter and end pieces might take even longer. Store in an airtight container and eat within a couple of days.

If you like the oily effect you get from shop-bought jars of sun-dried tomatoes, you can store your homemade ones in jars of olive oil with a few leaves of basil and a couple cloves of garlic. Marinate for at least a day, and add to salads.

ZACHARY'S SNACK

No equipment needed • 2 minutes

*This couldn't be simpler, and makes a wonderful nibble. I've given a
basic amount—you can multiply it up to feed a family or even a party!
It's good for school lunches instead of chips.*

1 tbsp broccoli bits (see page 166)

1 tbsp sprouted sunflower and pumpkin seeds (see below)

1 tbsp dulse flakes

1 tbsp lentil or mung sprouts

Crumble the broccoli bits so they're the same size as the seeds. It's always
best to soak seeds first to activate the enzymes—if you want to give them a
crunch back, dehydrate them for a bit after soaking them. Mix the lot
together and munch, for the most nutritious snack you're ever going to
come across. This doesn't really store well; the bits start to go soggy. It's
best to make only as much as you need, and eat it right away.

*We make this with Raw Living "Sunseeds," which is a mix
of sunflower and pumpkin seeds ready sprouted,
marinated in tamari and dehydrated.*

CEREAL

Dehydrator • 5 minutes (4–8 hours soaking,
3 days sprouting, 12 hours dehydrating)

*For a long time, we had fruit for breakfast, either a pudding or a
smoothie. But as we detoxified, we noticed more and more the effect
this early morning sugar hit had on our bodies and began to search
for an alternative. This (or raw oatmeal) is what the boys
have for their breakfast most mornings.*

1 oz/30 g raisins

1 oz/30 g pumpkin or sunflower seeds

4 oz/120 g buckwheat bits (see below)

1 tsp agave syrup

1 tbsp flax oil

1 tsp lecithin granules

Soak the raisins and seeds for at least 4 hours. We put ours in to soak just before we go to bed, ready for the morning. Drain them and put them in a mixing bowl with all the other ingredients. Give them a good stir round, so the agave and oil are evenly coating the cereal. Divide into bowls and serve.

Variations:

· You can substitute just about any dried fruit, nuts, or seeds in this that you like.

· You can substitute tahini or nut butter for the oil.

· You can add 1 tbsp carob powder for carob cereal.

· On special occasions you can add 2 tbsp cacao nibs and 2 tbsp goji berries for a super-food cereal!

To make the buckwheat bits, sprout some buckwheat groats for about three days, and then dry them in the dehydrator for 12 hours: 10 oz (300 g) unsoaked buckwheat will make about 15 oz (450 g) of crunchy bits (or 6 servings of cereal). Store in an airtight container, and they will keep for a good couple of months.

QUICKLES

No equipment needed • 5 minutes

Pickles for cheats! I've tried to make sauerkraut a handful of times, but it's yet to work, and there are a few good raw ones available on the market, so it doesn't seem worth the bother. But these are so easy, and surprisingly good.

$\frac{1}{2}$ cucumber or 2 onions

8 fl oz/250 ml apple cider vinegar

Chop the cucumber or onion into small chunks. Put in a jar of vinegar and store in the fridge. Eat the next day (will keep for a few weeks). It's that easy!

> *I use the organic apple cider vinegar that's left when we've finished a jar of gherkins. You can usually use it twice before you have to throw it out.*

PLANTAIN CHIPS

Food processor, dehydrator • 10 minutes (12 hours dehydrating)

Plantains are a staple food in many parts of Africa and Asia and can often be picked up very cheaply in markets. Green plantain is usually used in entrees; yellow plantain is ripe and more like bananas. Green plantains work better for chip making as they are firmer and go crunchier.

3 plantains

2 tbsp olive oil

Fine slice the plantains in a food processor or salad slicer. Transfer them in a bowl and coat them in oil—add a little chili powder if you like a bit of heat. Arrange them over two drying trays, separating them out as much as possible. Dry for 12 hours. Store in an airtight container and eat as soon as possible—they won't go off quickly, but they will soften and lose their crunch.

> *There are some lovely gourmet plantain chips on the market; they aren't raw, but they're often a much healthier alternative to potato chips.*

PUDDINGS

With raw foods you can both have your cake and eat it. I'm here to tell you that this is a pudding revolution! Raw desserts taste amazing—they can be just as fat laden and syrupy sweet as your heart desires. But because we are using healthy fats that the body loves and nutritious sweeteners that don't destabilize blood sugar levels, you can eat as much of them as you like. In fact, some of them are so good you can eat them for breakfast, lunch, and dinner and feel super energized! I have a passion for puddings—it gives me great joy to feed pudding to people at every possible opportunity.

CAROB COCONUT PUDDING

Blender

15 minutes (4–8 hours soaking)

Serves 4

It's just a guess, but I think you could probably live on this, it contains so much nutrition. Hemp seeds are one of my favorite foods; they contain nearly everything the body needs to live on. Whole hemp seeds haven't been processed so they are a better source of nutrition, but the shells have quite a strong taste and crunchy texture that some people find unpalatable. For this reason, hulled seeds are very popular as they have a lovely creamy taste. You can use whichever you prefer in this recipe.

1 fresh coconut

4 bananas, peeled and chopped

4 oz/120 g pitted fresh dates

2 oz/60 g carob powder

2 lemons, juiced

8 fl oz/250 ml water

2 oz/60 g hemp seeds, soaked 4–8 hours

Remove the flesh from the coconut shell (see page 84). Put the bananas, dates, carob powder, lemon juice, and water in the blender, and blend to a liquid. Then add the hemp seeds and coconut pieces, and blend for a few minutes until you have a cream. If you haven't got a high-powered blender, you may need to grate the coconut in the food processor first, to make it easier for your machine. Serve within 24 hours and store in the fridge; fresh coconut doesn't keep well.

Banana plants are part of the same family as lilies and orchids.

BREAKFAST PUDDING

Blender

5 minutes (8–12 hours soaking)

Serves 2

Here is a light but filling breakfast to set you up for the day. The flax oil and lecithin give the pudding a real creaminess, as well as being a valuable source of nutrition. Lecithin helps with the absorption of fats so you can get the most out of those all-important essential fatty acids in the flax oil.

2 oz/60 g sesame seeds, soaked 8–12 hours

1 oz/30 g raisins, soaked 8–12 hours

2 apples

1 banana

1 tbsp flax oil

1 tbsp lecithin granules

Soak your sesame seeds and raisins overnight. Prepare the apples and banana for the blender by removing skins, stems, seeds, and so on. Pop all your ingredients in the blender and whiz up to a smooth puree. It's best eaten the same day.

If you've got any leftovers, you can spread the mixture onto a dehydrator sheet and dry it until it turns into a chewy snack.

GORGEOUS GOJI PUDDING

Blender

10 minutes (2 hours soaking)

Serves 2

*Wow! This bright orange pudding is sure to give you a lift. Goji berries
are a super food, the most nutrient-dense fruit on the planet.*

2 oz/60 g goji berries, soaked 2 hours

1 avocado

1 banana

1 medjool date, pitted

1 tbsp agave nectar

Soak the gojis in just enough water to cover them. When they've plumped
up, drink the soaking water—it's yummy. Slice the avocado in half, remove
the stone, and using a spoon, scoop the flesh out into the blender. Put the
berries in the blender along with the banana, peeled and broken into
chunks, the date, and the agave. Blend to a cream. If your blender isn't
strong enough, add a little water until it will keep going. It's best eaten the
same day.

*Goji berries are fairly recent health heroes in the West. They are
very common in Chinese cuisine, where they have been eaten
for thousands of years and are also used medicinally.*

BEST EVER CHOCOLATE PUDDING

Blender

5 minutes

Serves 2

*This is probably one of the most popular raw food desserts. If you're new
to raw foods, you'll be amazed at how avocado can form the base of one
of the most luscious raw puddings around. If you're an experienced
raw fooder, you've probably had chocolate pudding many times.
It's my favorite sweet treat, and so easy to prepare—ready in
minutes with no presoaking or dehydrating necessary.*

1 oz/30 g ground cacao nibs

1 large avocado

1 banana

1 medjool date

1 tbsp agave nectar

1 tbsp hemp oil

1 oz/30 g carob powder

Grind your cacao in a coffee grinder or high-powered blender. Slice the
avocado in half, remove the pit, scoop out the flesh with a spoon, and put
it straight into the blender. Peel the banana, break into quarters, and add
to the blender. Remove the stone from the date and pop it in the jug too.
Add the remaining ingredients. If you haven't got cacao, you can use double
carob powder instead; it won't give you the same chocolate hit, but it will
taste nearly as divine. Turn the blender on and start whizzing. If your blender
is having difficulties, you can add some water until it starts turning over.
Keep it turning for a minute to make sure it's really smooth and creamy.
Spoon out into two serving bowls; decorate with carob chips or goji berries if
you fancy. Or add a tablespoon of maca powder for a lover's pudding!

*Cacao, the raw chocolate bean, is causing a revolution
in the raw food world and beyond. Everyone loves
the chocolate that loves you back!*

TOFFEE CREAM

Blender

5 minutes (8–12 hours soaking)

Serves 4

This is a rich gooey dessert that goes brilliantly with fresh berries
in the summer or sliced apples and pears in the autumn.

7 oz/200 g cashews, soaked 8–12 hours

2 oz/60 g carob powder

4 tbsp olive oil

2 tbsp agave nectar

8 fl oz/250 ml water

Soak your cashews in advance. Put all the ingredients together in a blender and blend to a smooth puree. It will keep in the fridge for about four days.

Instead of cashews, you can substitute hulled hemp seeds,
macadamias, or pine nuts if you prefer.

CAN'T BETA IT

Blender • 5 minutes (12 hours freezing, 1 hour presoaking)

Serves 2

Apricots and goji berries are both excellent sources of beta-carotene (vitamin A). This is a beautiful, bright and breezy summery pudding.

2 bananas, frozen 12 hours

2 oz/60 g goji berries, soaked 1 hour

8 fresh apricots

Peel your bananas, break them into small chunks, and put them in a bag or tub in the freezer for at least 12 hours. It isn't essential to use frozen bananas, but you get a much thicker pudding if you do. Soak the gojis for about an hour and then drain (drink the soak water, it's gorgeous!). Remove the stones from the apricots, and put the flesh in the blender along with the gojis and bananas. Blend until there are no chunks of banana left. Serve immediately.

A single apricot contains about 20 percent of the RDA for vitamin A, so this pudding should easily satisfy your daily requirement.

HEMP ICE CREAM

Ice-cream maker, blender • 5 minutes (8–12 hours soaking, 20 minutes freezing)

Serves 4

You need an ice-cream maker for these ice-cream recipes, but it is so worth the investment for an amazing variety of raw ice creams. Once you have tried them, you will be hooked—we have them every week throughout the summer.

8 oz/250 g whole hemp seeds, soaked 8–12 hours

16 fl oz/500 ml water

4 oz/120 g fresh dates

4 tbsp olive oil

Presoak the hemp seeds. Blend all the ingredients to a cream. Pour into the ice-cream maker and proceed according to the manufacturer's instructions. You should get fantastic results in less than half an hour.

Variation: replace the hemp seeds with pumpkin seeds
for a green ice cream.

HALVA ICE CREAM

Ice-cream maker, blender • 5 minutes (8–12 hours soaking,
20 minutes freezing) • Serves 4

We love halva! We used to be addicted to vegan halva made with grape juice, but it's not raw. Plus, too much of those cooked sesame seeds aren't health giving and start to clog you up. This, on the other hand, is guilt-free!

14 oz/400 g sesame seeds, soaked 8–12 hours

4 oz/120 g pitted fresh dates

16 fl oz/500 ml water

1 vanilla pod

4 oz/120 g raisins

Soak your sesame seeds in advance. Blend the sesame seeds, dates, water, and vanilla to a thick cream, so there are no seedy bits or fragments of pod left. Stir in the raisins by hand. Pour into your ice-cream maker and proceed according to the manufacturer's instructions. It usually takes about 20 minutes to make heavenly raw ice cream.

Apparently, there is a Greek saying, Ante re halva!, which translates as "Get lost, halva!" and is used to offend someone by implying they are effeminate!

CAROB ICE CREAM

Ice-cream maker, blender

5 minutes (8–12 hours soaking,
about 20 minutes freezing)

Serves 6

*If you can track down some lúcuma powder, substitute it for the carob in
this recipe. Lúcuma is a Peruvian fruit that has a beautiful rich flavor,
and is Peru's most popular choice for adding to ice cream.*

8 oz/250 g sunflower seeds, soaked 8–12 hours

4 tbsp olive oil

3 oz/90 g carob powder

4 oz/120 g pitted fresh dates

27 fl oz/750 ml water

1 tbsp cinnamon

Soak your sunflower seeds in advance. Blend everything together for a few
minutes to a runny cream. Pour into your ice-cream maker, and proceed
according to the manufacturer's instructions. Serve with strawberries on a
hot summer's day.

*The tallest recorded sunflower grew to 40 feet.
Sunflowers are heliotropic, that is, as the sun moves
across the sky in a day, the flower head turns to face
the sun and follows it from east to west.*

FRUIT KEBABS

Cocktail sticks or barbecue skewers

10 minutes

These are great for children to make and enjoy, although they will need supervision. Smaller children will be happy with cocktail sticks; if you are making them for older children (or adults!), barbecue skewers may be preferable. Serve with a chocolate sauce or nut cream for dipping like a fondue.

Selection of firm fresh fruits
(such as apple, pear, mango, pineapple, grapes)
Selection of dried fruits
(such as lexia raisins, dates, apricots)

I haven't given quantities as it really depends on your taste and imagination. Gather together a selection of your favorite fruits and dried fruits; three different fruits and two different dried fruits works well. Prepare them so that you have cubes, about the size of a grape, ready to pierce on your skewer or cocktail stick. Grapes you can leave whole. Lexia raisins are extra-large raisins; you can leave these whole too. Dates or apricots can be halved.

Once your fruit is ready, you can call the children to come and help you. They love choosing for themselves what to put on each stick. It's best to have a lot more fresh fruit than dried fruit to avoid a sugar overload. Arrange the sticks on a plate or serving dish.

For parties, cut a Galia melon in half and skewer the kebabs into the skin to make a hedgehog!

EASTER APPLES

Blender • 30 minutes (4–8 hours soaking) • Serves 4

This is my raw approximation of cream eggs.
How will you eat yours?

4 oz/120 g sesame seeds, soaked 4–8 hours

4 small apples

2 bananas

4 oz/120 g fresh dates

2 oz/60 g carob powder

1 tbsp grain coffee

1 vanilla pod

Soak your sesame seeds in advance. Chop the lids off the apples, setting them aside, and scoop out the core. Hollow them out as if you were making Halloween pumpkins, so you're making an apple shell, ready to fill with the carob mixture. Ideally you want about $\frac{1}{2}$ inch apple flesh round the edge. Put the center flesh aside for another use. Put all the ingredients apart from the apples in the blender, and blend to a puree. Fill each apple with the mixture and pop the lids back on. Serve immediately.

Variation: if you have cacao nibs, you can add 2 oz (50 g) and omit the grain coffee.

GOJI AND MACADAMIA MINCEMEAT MESS

Blender • 1 hour • Serves 8

This was Jamie Oliver's idea. The English dessert Eton mess is traditionally made with strawberries, cream, and meringues— he did a Christmas version with mincemeat. This is my raw version with mincemeat, cream, and clementines.

4 clementines

1 tbsp goji berries

Mincemeat

1 lemon

1 orange

12 oz/360 g grated apple

4 oz/120 g lexia raisins

4 oz/120 g mixed raisins

4 oz/120 g goji berries

2 oz/60 g chopped dates

1 tbsp ground cinnamon

1 tsp ground ginger

Pinch ground nutmeg

Pinch ground cloves

2 tbsp olive oil

1 tbsp agave syrup

1 tbsp molasses

1 tsp miso

Macadamia cream

11 oz/330 g macadamia nuts

4 oz/120 g dates

1 vanilla pod

2 tbsp olive oil

16 fl oz/500 ml water

1. Peel the clementines and separate the segments; remove the seeds. Set the clementines and goji berries aside while preparing the mincemeat and macadamia cream.

2. To make the mincemeat: Juice the lemon and the orange, and grate the rind. Using a wooden spoon, combine all the ingredients together in a large bowl, so it's nice and evenly mixed.

3. To make the macadamia cream: Put everything in the blender and whiz to a thick cream.

4. To assemble: In a large glass dish, make a bottom layer with half the mincemeat. Cover with a layer of cream, and dot with clementines. Use the remaining mincemeat for another layer, top with cream again (you don't need to use all of this rich cream—you may find yourself with a few spoons leftover that you can refrigerate for another day or dehydrate for a sweet snack). Finish with the clementines, arranging them artfully over the top. Sprinkle with the remaining goji berries for decoration.

Raisins are unique in that they are the only dried fruit not to bear the same name as the fresh fruit—do you ever hear of people snacking on dried grapes?!

CHRISTMAS ICED BOMBE

Food processor or blender
40 minutes (24 hours freezing, 90 minutes defrosting)
Serves 12

This one is adapted from a supermarket recipe card. I've always loved the combination of mincemeat and ice cream, and this dish seems a perfect marriage. It's very easy to do and keeps for ages in the freezer.

8 bananas

Mincemeat

1 lemon

1 orange

12 oz/360 g grated apple

4 oz/120 g lexia raisins

4 oz/120 g mixed raisins

4 oz/120 g goji berries

2 oz/60 g chopped dates

1 tbsp ground cinnamon

1 tsp ground ginger

Pinch ground nutmeg

Pinch ground cloves

2 tbsp olive oil

1 tbsp agave syrup

1 tbsp molasses

1 tsp miso

1. Peel, chop, and blend the bananas to a lump-free liquid. Set aside.

2. To make the mincemeat: Juice the lemon and the orange, and grate the rind. Using a wooden spoon, combine all the ingredients together in a large bowl, so it's nice and evenly mixed.

3. Stir the bananas into the mincemeat in a big bowl. Line a large Pyrex bowl with plastic wrap (you may need two sheets, one going up each side). Fill the bowl with the mincemeat and banana mixture, and place in the freezer for 24 hours. Remove from the freezer 90 minutes before you're ready to eat it. After an hour at room temperature, it should be defrosted enough that you can turn the bowl upside down onto a plate and it will loosen. Remove the plastic wrap, and leave for a further 20–30 minutes to soften.

4. If there are any leftovers, slice them up, wrap them individually, and store in the freezer. Then they just need 20–30 minutes defrosting time.

If you don't want to use goji berries, or can't get them, you can omit them and just double the amount of mixed raisins.

TRIFLE

Blender • I hour (8–12 hours soaking) • Serves 8

A must at Christmas. This is based around four different recipes, put together in one feast of a dessert.

Layer 1: fruit in banana jelly

2 kiwi fruit

8 oz/250 g seedless grapes

2 satsumas

1 lemon

2 bananas

$\frac{1}{2}$ tbsp psyllium husk powder

Layer 2: apple pudding

1 lb/500 g apples

4 oz/120 g raisins, soaked 4–8 hours

1 tsp cinnamon

Layer 3: chocolate pudding

1 avocado

1 banana

2 oz/60 g pitted fresh dates

1 tbsp carob powder

Layer 4: cashew cream

4 oz/120 g cashews, soaked 8–12 hours

1 tbsp olive oil

2 tbsp agave nectar

1 vanilla pod

4 tbsp water

Layer 5: topping

3 pieces dried mango

3 pieces dried pineapple

1 tbsp goji berries

1 tbsp cacao nibs

1. Find a big serving dish, preferably glass or Pyrex, so you can see all the layers through it once it's done. It needs to be quite deep—the one I use is about 3 inches deep and $8\frac{1}{2}$ inches in diameter. To begin, prepare the fruit. Peel the kiwi; slice each into about 16 pieces. Remove the grapes from the stem; if they are large, slice them in half. Peel the satsumas and separate the segments. Put them all together in a mixing bowl. Juice the lemon, and put it in the blender with the bananas, peeled and broken up. Blend until there are no lumps of banana left, and then add the psyllium. Blend for a further minute, until the psyllium is mixed through. Pour this mixture over the fruit pieces, and stir so they are coated evenly. Spoon the mixture into the trifle dish, flattening it out on top.

2. Clean out the blender, ready to make the apple pudding. Chop the apples, and remove the cores. Put them in the blender and puree. Add the soaked raisins and cinnamon, and puree again. Once the raisins have completely disappeared into the mixture, it's ready. Spoon it out straight into your serving dish, covering the fruit layer completely.

3. Next is my favorite, the chocolate pudding! Clean the blender out once more. Peel and break the banana, scoop out the avocado flesh, and add them both to the blender with the dates and the carob. If it won't blend nicely, you can add a little water to help it along. Once it's all amalgamated, spoon it out on top of the apple layer, flattening the top off nicely.

4. Finally for the blender is cashew cream. Make sure you've cleaned the blender properly, or the carob will turn your cream brown. Put the cashews, olive oil, agave, vanilla, and water in the blender and whiz away. You may need to add more water—up to 4 tablespoons—more. Keep it running for a few minutes until you have a thick but smooth cream—if it's granular, add a little more water and blend some more. Spoon it onto the carob pudding, being careful not to let any of the brown mix into the white.

5. Now for the topping: Using scissors cut the mango and pineapple pieces into tiny bits. Sprinkle them over the cream with the goji berries and cacao for a "hundreds and thousands" effect. There you have it—a beautiful creation that tastes as good as it looks.

You can make this into knickerbocker glory (very elaborate
sundae) by omitting the bottom "jelly" layer, and serving
the remaining four layers heaped into tall glasses.

CAKES

I find that making cakes is just as much fun as eating them. There's something very therapeutic about assembling all these gorgeous ingredients with their enticing aromas and then creating a beautiful offering that you know your friends and family are going to love when you share it with them. And of course, there's all that taste testing you have to do along the way! None of these cakes can be knocked out in a few minutes, but they're still considerably simpler to make than most conventional cooked cakes. The best thing about raw cake making is you don't have to worry too much if something goes wrong in preparation; you don't have to concern yourself with things not rising or burning. However it turns out, if it ends up being a little sloppy or misshapen, it's still going to taste amazing! Raw cakes are a revelation—again, we can have our cake and eat it too!

LEMON TART

Food processor, blender

30 minutes (2 hours setting)

Serves 8

*We were visiting my friend Emma, who is a very good vegan cake-maker
(and the editor of the British natural parenting magazine Juno), and she
served us some vegan lemon tart, which inspired my raw version. The carob
crust makes a wonderfully rich contrast to the sharpness of the lemons.*

Pie Crust

7 oz/200 g almonds

7 oz/200 g raisins

2 tbsp carob powder

Filling

8 lemons

8 oz/250 g pitted fresh dates

3 bananas

1 tbsp psyllium

1. To make the pie crust: Grind the almonds in a coffee grinder or high-powered blender. Mash the raisins in a food processor until they become a ball. Add the almonds and the carob powder to the food processor and process until they form a smooth ball together. You may need to add a drop or two of water to make it firm. Press this mixture into an 8 inch pie tin, enough to cover the base and about $\frac{3}{4}$ inch up the sides. Set aside.

2. To make the filling: Peel the lemons and remove the seeds. Put the flesh in the blender with the dates and bananas. Blend to a liquid puree. Add the psyllium and blend some more. Immediately transfer the filling into the crust.

3. Leave to set for a few hours in the refrigerator.

*Did you know a single lemon provides you with
40 percent RDA of vitamin C?*

BANANA CRÈME PIE

Food processor, blender • 30 minutes (8–12 hours soaking,
2 hours setting) • Serves 12

*This makes a lovely treat, but it's very rich so you can't eat too much
of it. Bananas and tahini are such a fabulous combination,
it really hits the spot.*

Pie Crust

7 oz/200 g almonds

7 oz/200 g raisins

2 tbsp carob powder

Filling

4 bananas

1 large apple

4 oz/120 g fresh dates

4 oz/120 g tahini

1 lemon, juiced

2 tsp vanilla extract

1 tbsp psyllium

1. To make the pie crust: Grind the almonds in a coffee grinder or high-powered blender. Mash the raisins in a food processor until they become a ball. Add the almonds and the carob powder to the food processor and process until they form a smooth ball together. You may need to add a drop or two of water to make it firm. Press this mixture into an 8 inch pie tin, enough to cover the base and about $\frac{3}{4}$ inch up the sides. Set aside.

2. To make the filling: Peel the bananas, break them into quarters, and put them in the blender. Chop the apple, discard the core, and put the apple pieces in the blender. Pit the dates and add them into the blender with the tahini, lemon juice, and vanilla extract. This will easily blend to a thick cream. When it's ready, pour in the psyllium and blend for a minute to make sure it's thoroughly worked in. Quickly pour it into the pie crust.

3. Leave to set in the fridge for a couple of hours before serving.

Bananas emit a natural gas called ethylene gas, which causes fruit to ripen. That's why placing ripe bananas next to hard fruit such as pears and avocados helps them to soften quicker. This is also why bananas should be stored separately from other fruit like oranges and lemons, not in the fruit bowl, unless you want them to get those soft moldy white patches!

APPLE CRÈME PIE

Food processor, blender • 30 minutes (8–12 hours soaking, 2 hours setting) • Serves 12

Research suggests that cinnamon might improve glucose control for diabetics; half a teaspoon of cinnamon a day has produced noticeable reductions in blood sugar levels. So when you add it to your desserts or oatmeal, not only are you improving the flavor, you could be helping to balance out your blood sugar!

Pie Crust

7 oz/200 g almonds

7 oz/200 g raisins

2 tbsp carob powder

Filling

8 apples

3 oz/90 g sesame seeds, soaked 8–12 hours

4 oz/120 g pitted fresh dates

1 tbsp cinnamon

1 lemon, juiced

1 tbsp psyllium

1. Soak the sesame seeds in advance.

2. To make the pie crust: Grind the almonds in a coffee grinder or high-powered blender. Mash the raisins in a food processor until they become

a ball. Add the almonds and the carob powder to the food processor and process until they form a smooth ball together. You may need to add a drop or two of water to make it firm. Press this mixture into an 8 inch pie tin, enough to cover the base and about $\frac{3}{4}$ inch up the sides. Set aside.

3. Chop and core the apples; put the pieces in the blender and blend to a puree. Add the sesame seeds, dates, cinnamon, and lemon juice, and blend again. When you're confident that everything is mixed up and there are no seedy bits left, add the psyllium. Blend for another minute. Pour into your crust and smooth out the top.

4. Leave in the fridge to set for a couple of hours.

Apples are grown in every state in the continental United States. Top-producing states include Washington, New York, Michigan, Pennsylvania, California, and Virginia. There are about 2,500 known varieties in the United States.

POPPY SEED TART

Food processor, blender
1 hour (8–12 hours soaking, 2 hours setting)
Serves 12

Poppy seeds are a wonderful addition to salads and sweet dishes: just a sprinkle adds crunchy texture and a light nutty flavor to dishes. They are a good source of calcium, but a mild opiate so don't eat too many! They are known for their narcotic properties and so are used as a traditional remedy for sleeplessness.

Pie Crust
4 oz/120 g sunflower seeds, soaked 1–2 hours
4 oz/120 g dates
1 tsp cinnamon

Filling

4 oz/120 g apricots, soaked 4 hours

2 oz/60 g dates

1 tsp vanilla extract

5 oz/150 g almonds, soaked 8–12 hours

4 bananas

4 fl oz/125 ml agave syrup

4 fl oz/125 ml olive oil

4 fl oz/125 ml water

2 tbsp psyllium

7 oz/200 g poppy seeds

1. To make the crust: Put the sunflower seeds in the food processor and process until they are as ground down as you can get them. Then add the dates and cinnamon, and process again until you have a dough. Press the mixture into a large pie dish to form a crust on the base and sides.

2. To make the filling: Clean out the food processor and put in the apricots, second lot of dates, and vanilla. Process until the apricots and dates are amalgamated, and press into your sunflower crust to make a layer on the bottom. Next in the blender put the almonds, bananas (peeled and broken into pieces), agave, olive oil, and water. Blend to a thick cream, then add the psyllium and blend for a further minute. By hand, stir in the poppy seeds, making sure you mix them evenly right through the mixture. The mixture should be quite solid. Spread it on the top of the apricot layer, quickly before it firms up completely.

3. Pop the tart in the fridge to set for a couple of hours.

Poppy seeds are banned in some countries, like Saudi Arabia, for instance, because of the morphine content. If you ate enough, you would test positive for opiates in a drug test!

THE BEST BIRTHDAY CAKE

Blender, dehydrator

1 hour (12–18 hours dehydrating)

Serves 12

This makes a dense sponge cake.

Cake

12 oz/360 g sprouted wheat grain
(see Sprouting, page 49)

3 oz/90 g carob powder

8 fl oz/250 ml olive oil

4 fl oz/125 ml agave nectar

4 fl oz/125 ml water

Filling

4 bananas

2 lemons

1 tbsp psyllium

Icing

7 oz/200 g tahini

2 bananas

2 oz/60 g carob powder

Decoration

1 tbsp lexia raisins

1 tbsp coconut chips

1 tbsp goji berries

1. Sprout the wheat three days in advance.

2. To make the cake: Put all the cake ingredients into the blender and whiz to a batter. Spread a third of the mixture on a dehydrator sheet in a large circle. Repeat with the rest of the batter, so you have three large circles that more or less fill each sheet. Dehydrate for 12–18 hours. Once cooled, slide one round onto a plate or cake tray, whatever you want to serve it on because you will not be able to move it again.

3. To make the filling, blend the bananas with the juice of the lemons and, once pureed, add the psyllium.

4. Working quickly before the psyllium sets, spoon half of the lemon mix onto the round. Put the second round on top, then repeat, so you have three layers—cake, lemon filling, cake, lemon filling, cake.

5. Then it's back to the blender to mix the tahini, bananas, and carob for the icing. This needs to be quite thick so it will stick to the sides of the cake. Using a knife, smooth it over the top and around the edge, so it looks like a proper iced cake.

6. Decorate with lexia raisins, coconut chips, and goji berries. Add the required number of candles and there you have it—a birthday cake fit for your little prince or princess!

Like currants and sultanas, lexias are just a different variety of dried grape. Fat and juicy, I have never seen organic ones for sale, but they make a lovely change from the standard variety in puddings, sweets, and chocolate.

CAROB TORTE

Food processor, blender

45 minutes

Serves 16

This is adapted from a recipe in Juliano's book, Raw: The Uncook
Book. *Fabulous as his recipe is, it is incredibly rich—
this is a toned-down version, but still very decadent.*

Crust

4 oz/120 g raisins

6 oz/180 g ground walnuts

1 tbsp cinnamon

Filling

8 oz/250 g fresh coconut pieces

14 oz/420 g pitted fresh dates

4 fl oz/125 ml agave nectar

8 oz/250 g ground cashews

7 oz/200 g carob powder

Icing

2 lemons

4 bananas

Topping

8 oz/250 g seasonal fruit

1. To make the crust: Mash the raisins in the food processor until they
form a solid mass. Add the nuts and cinnamon, and process until the nuts
and raisins are completely mixed together. Press into a pie dish, just lining
the base, not the sides.

2. To make the filling: Clean the food processor and put the coconut
pieces in. Process until it's evenly broken down into small pieces, the size of
raisins or rice grains. Remove from the food processor and put in a large
mixing bowl. Process the dates until they form a ball. With the machine
running, gradually add the agave to the dates. Once it's all mixed together,

add to the mixing bowl with your coconut chips, ground cashews, and carob powder. With a wooden spoon, mix everything together until the mixture is stiff. Spoon it into your pie dish, on top of the crust.

3. To make the icing: Juice the lemons, and pour the juice in the blender with the bananas, peeled and broken into pieces. Blend until there are no lumps of banana left. Pour this over your torte.

4. Finally, arrange your fruit on top: mixed berries are great in the summer, or clementine segments in the winter. You can serve it right away, or keep it in the fridge for up to a week.

Carob pods are so plentiful in southern Spain, farmers do not know what to do with them and use them as animal feed.

ETHAN'S CAKE

Food processor, blender

45 minutes (2 hours setting)

Serves 12

Ethan invented this recipe for his fourth birthday. His birthday is in January, so there's not much fruit around, and this is what he came up with. It sounds pretty plain, but the flavors do amazing things together, and it actually turned out to be one of our favorite cakes.

Crust

5 oz/150 g ground almonds

4 oz/120 g pitted fresh dates

1 tbsp carob powder

Filling

2 large or 3 small apples

2 large or 3 small pears

2 lemons

4 bananas

1 tbsp psyllium husk powder

4 oz/120 g lexia raisins

1. To prepare the crust: Grind the almonds in a coffee grinder or high-powered blender. Mash the dates in the food processor. Once they've formed a sticky mass, add the carob and the almonds and process again until it's all mixed together in a gorgeous brown goo. Press it into the cake tin, at the base and up the sides, and try not to lick your fingers until you've finished.

2. To make the filling: Prepare the apples and pears by removing the cores and chopping them so they'll fit in the chute of your food processor. Using the fine-slicing blade, slice the apples and pears and put them in a mixing bowl. Juice the lemons, and add to the blender with the bananas. Blend until there are no lumps left. Add the psyllium, and blend for another minute. Pour it into the bowl with the apples and pears. Add the raisins and stir it up so the fruit is well mixed.

3. To assemble, spoon the filling into your crust, flatten the top, and leave to set in the fridge for a couple of hours.

Pears top the list of foods that people are least likely to be allergic to. I once lived with a guy named Mike who was allergic to practically everything but pears, rice, and lamb. Pears make a great first food for babies because they are hypoallergenic.

REUBEN'S CAKE

Food processor, blender

45 minutes

Serves 12

Not to be outdone, here's the recipe Reuben came up with for his birthday that same year. He has a summer birthday, so we made the most of the wonderful seasonal berries. As this cake's quite solid, you aren't restricted to using a cake tin. You can make it on a tray or large plate, and mold it into whatever shape you wish—a heart or a star. Reuben had a number seven because it was his seventh birthday.

Base

4 oz/120 g ground sunflower seeds

4 oz/120 g ground hemp seeds

4 oz/120 g raisins

2 oz/60 g carob powder

Layer 1

1 large mango

2 nectarines

1 lemon, juiced

1 tbsp psyllium husk powder

Layer 2

4 oz/120 g pitted fresh dates

4 oz/120 g ground cashews

Layer 3

1 lb/500 g strawberries

8 oz/250 g raspberries

8 oz/250 g blueberries

1. To make the base, grind the sunflower seeds and hemp seeds in a coffee grinder or high-powered blender. Mash the raisins in the food processor. Then add the sunflower seeds and hemp seeds and process until they are evenly mixed. Next add the carob powder and process again. If it doesn't stick together, you may want to add a few drops of water. Press it down flat onto your serving tray.

2. To make the first layer: Remove the mango flesh from the stone, and peel off the skins. Put the flesh in the blender, along with the nectarines, pitted and chopped, and lemon juice. The resulting mixture will be quite liquid. Add the psyllium and blend again. Leave it to one side for a few minutes so it starts to thicken. Once it's gone to jelly, spoon it onto the seed base.

3. To make the second layer: Mash the dates in the food processor. Once they're a solid mass, add the cashews and combine. Spread this layer on top of your now set jelly layer.

4. Finally, press the berries into the cake, completely covering the top and sides. The result is a beautiful berry feast—too good for anyone to turn down!

There are hundreds of varieties of mango grown worldwide—
India is the main producer.

CHOCOLATE CAKE

Juicer, blender, dehydrator

45 minutes (24 hours dehydrating)

Serves 8

On one of the raw Internet chat groups, someone posted a message about raw chocolate cake, and I've never seen such a response. People were clamoring for the recipe. There wasn't one, so I thought I'd better try and work one out. Out of all the cakes, this is by far my favorite, reminiscent of the Victoria sponges I grew up on. I originally wrote the recipe with carob, but since then the wondrous cacao bean has appeared on the scene, so now we can have our chocolate cake and eat it too!

Cake

6 oz/180 g sprouted wheat
(see Sprouting, page 49)

5 oz/150 g pitted fresh dates

4 oz/120 g cacao nibs

4 fl oz/125 ml olive oil

Filling

1 banana

1 avocado

2 tbsp agave nectar

2 tbsp raw chocolate powder

1. To make the cake: You really need a juicer for this, as nothing else will mash up the wheat sprouts. Put the sprouts through with the blank plate on, followed by the dates and the cacao nibs if you're using them. In a large mixing bowl, knead the sprouts, dates, cacao, and olive oil all together. Your hands are really the best tool for getting everything thoroughly mixed here. When it's done, divide the mixture into two halves. On drying trays, shape into rounds about 2 inches deep and 8 inches in diameter. Dehydrate for 12 hours. Take two clean drying trays, and flip the cakes over to make sure they dry on the other side. Dehydrate for a further 12 hours.

2. To make the filling: When the cakes are done, you're ready to make the filling. Peel the banana, break it into pieces, and put it in the blender. Scoop out the avocado flesh, and add that to the blender along with the agave and raw chocolate. Blend up to a cream—add a little water if you're having difficulty.

3. To assemble: Slide one of your cakes onto a serving plate. Spoon the cream on top, nice and thick. Slide the second cake on top, and it's ready to eat.

If you like this, you'll like Shazzie and David Wolfe's book
Naked Chocolate, which as well as being interesting reading on
the history and nutritional properties of raw chocolate
is bursting with mouth-watering recipes.

COCONUT TORTE

Food processor, blender
45 minutes (2 hours setting)
Serves 12

This was a real favorite in our house for a while. It's rich and yet
somehow light at the same time. Coconut is wonderfully health giving—
we eat a lot of it. Full of lauric acid, a highly beneficial fatty acid,
it balances the metabolism and so it's a fat that you can
eat a lot of without putting on weight.

Base
6 oz/180 g ground walnuts
2 fresh coconuts
4 oz/120 g raisins
1 tbsp cinnamon

Filling

3 oz/90 g carob powder

8 oz/250 g pitted fresh dates

2 tsp tamari

2 tbsp grain coffee

4 fl oz/125 ml olive oil

4 fl oz/125 ml agave nectar

8 fl oz/250 ml water

Topping

8 oz/250 g raspberries

1. To make the base: Grind the walnuts in a coffee grinder or high-powered blender. Extract the coconut meat from the shell (see page 84). Take the walnuts, raisins, cinnamon, and 1 cup of coconut pieces. Mash the raisins in the food processor until you have a solid mass. Then add the coconut flesh, and grind some more. Once all the coconut's worked in, add the ground walnuts and cinnamon, and process until everything is evenly combined. Press the mixture into your pie dish, making just a flat layer on the bottom.

2. To make the filling: Put the remaining coconut meat, carob, dates, tamari, grain coffee, olive oil, agave, and water in the blender. You should have enough liquid that it doesn't have a problem turning over. If you have a standard blender, you might have a bit of a problem; you might try mashing the dates and coconut in the food processor first. You don't want to add any more water or it will be too runny. The result should be a very thick, slightly granular cream.

3. To assemble: Spoon the filling into your pie dish, level out the top, and decorate with the fresh raspberries. Leave to set for an hour or two before serving.

In southern Thailand, a type of monkey called the pig-tailed macaque is trained to harvest the coconuts from the palms, and competitions are held to find the fastest harvester.

MALT LOAF

Blender, dehydrator

20 minutes (8–12 hours soaking, 24 hours dehydrating)

Serves 8

*At the Tree of Life Rejuvenation Center in Arizona, they make breads
and loaves based on flaxseeds. When I tried one of their recipes,
I found it very reminiscent of malt loaf. This is my adaptation—
it's delightfully squidgy and substantial without being sickly.*

2 oz/60 g figs, soaked 4–8 hours

2 oz/60 g apricots, soaked 4–8 hours

6 oz/180 g walnuts, soaked 8–12 hours

4 oz/120 g almonds, soaked 8–12 hours

1 tbsp cinnamon

1 tbsp mixed spice

4 tbsp yacon syrup or molasses

10 oz/300 g ground flaxseeds

Soak your figs, apricots, walnuts, and almonds in advance. When they're
ready, drain them off. You should discard the soak water from the nuts, but
you can drink the water from the dried fruit (it's delicious). Put all the
ingredients except the flaxseeds in the blender. The nuts and dried fruits
should have absorbed enough water to make the mixture runny enough to
blend. Spoon the mixture out into a mixing bowl and stir in the flaxseeds
with a spoon. They will stiffen the mixture considerably. Transfer it to a
drying tray, and mold it into a loaf shape, about 2 inches high (no taller, or
it won't dry through properly). Dry for 12 hours, then turn it over so the
bottom side gets done too, and dry for a further 12 hours. Serve with raw
nut butter for a snack.

*The Tree of Life center, which was founded in 1993 by Dr.
Gabriel Cousens, has become one of the foremost focal points
for raw food teaching in the world. The center is set on 182
acres of land and is home to people from over 100 nations.*

ICE-CREAM LAYER CAKE

Blender, dehydrator, ice-cream maker

40 minutes (sprouting time, 8–12 hours soaking,
18 hours dehydrating)

Serves 12–16

This makes a perfect summer birthday cake.

Cake layer

10 oz/300 g sprouted buckwheat
(see Sprouting, page 49)

3 oz/90 g carob powder
or 4 oz/120 g ground cacao nibs

2 tbsp agave nectar

8 fl oz/250 ml water

Ice-cream layer

7 oz/200 g cashews, soaked 8–12 hours

8 fresh dates, pitted

1 tbsp vanilla extract

8 fl oz/250 ml water

Icing

2 tbsp almond butter

2 tbsp agave nectar

1 tbsp carob powder

Decoration

2 tbsp goji berries

3 oz/90 g fresh berries if they're in season

1. Sprout the buckwheat two or three days in advance. Soak the cashews
overnight.

2. To make the cake layer: Put all the cake ingredients in the blender and
blend to a cream. Spoon it out onto three drying trays and shape into large
circles, which should each take up most of the tray. The important thing is

that they are more or less the same size, because you are going to stack them one on top of the other. Dry the rounds for 12 hours, then flip over (hold a second, clean tray on top and then turn the rounds upside down, and remove the first tray). Dry for another 6 hours.

3. To make the ice-cream layer: Blend all the ice-cream ingredients together to a cream and pour into your ice-cream maker. Mine takes about 20 minutes of churning to turn nut cream into ice cream. It needs to be quite solid but still spreadable.

4. To assemble: Slide a cake layer onto a large plate, and spoon half the ice cream over the top to make a nice thick layer, spreading it right to the edge. Slide the second cake layer on top, and cover that with the remaining ice cream. Slide the third cake layer on top.

5. Make the icing by mixing the almond butter, agave, and carob in a bowl with a spoon. If it's not runny enough to spread, add water. Using a knife or a spoon, spread it thinly over the top of the cake.

6. Decorate with goji berries or whatever fruit is in season—strawberries are a winner. Eat immediately. Store leftovers in the freezer—to eat, remove 20 minutes before you're ready to allow it to defrost and soften a little so you can cut yourself a slice.

Americans eat the most ice cream of any nation in the world—
6 gallons a year on average.

COOKIES

In this section we celebrate the cookies you can eat as many of as you like without worrying about putting on weight, or clogging up your arteries, or getting a sugar overdose. Eating raw cookies is such a joy—not only are you feeding your body nutrient-dense goodies it loves, you are liberating your mind too! I was brought up almost to be scared of cookies. They were always around, part of the daily diet but to be monitored and carefully controlled for fear of going over my calorie count for the day, or getting pimples, or spoiling my appetite for dinner. To be able to eat as many sweet snacks as your heart desires without a trace of guilt is a wonderful experience everyone deserves to have. Make a batch, share them with your friends, and spread the joy!

Strawberry Shortcake

Blender, dehydrator
5 minutes (8–12 hours presoaking, 24 hours dehydrating)
Makes 25 cookies

These are lovely melt-in-the-mouth summer cookies for when strawberries are in season. You can substitute any berry for the strawberries—blueberries and raspberries are gorgeous.

10 oz/300 g Brazil nuts, presoaked 8–12 hours
7 oz/200 g strawberries
2 oz/60 g pitted dates
4 tbsp olive oil
4–8 fl oz/125–250 ml water
2 tsp cinnamon

Soak your Brazil nuts in advance. Dice the strawberries into tiny pieces, about the size of raisins. Mix everything else in the blender and puree so there are no bits of nut left. Use as little water as possible, or your cookies will be too soggy. Stir in the berries by hand. Spread the mixture onto a dehydrating tray. Dry for 12 hours, and then score into about 25 cookies (5 across by 5 down). Turn and dry for another 12 hours. Stored in an airtight tin in the fridge, they will keep for up to a week.

If you have the time and inclination, these cookies are even better when the berries are dried first. Dice them, spread them on a tray, and dry for 6–12 hours. Then add the dried berries into the mix, so you end up with a chewier berry in the finished cookie.

Lovely Biscuits

Blender, dehydrator
15 minutes (8–12 hours presoaking, 16 hours dehydrating)
Makes about 40 cookies

The great thing about these is they are sweet without containing too much sugary stuff. Stevia is an herb that is 30–100 times sweeter than sugar! So a few drops of it will do in your cakes and cookies instead of any other sweetener. If you taste it straight from the bottle or packet, it's not very nice, like strong molasses; but in a recipe it is one of the healthiest and least sickly sweeteners you can find.

5 oz/150 g Brazil nuts, soaked 8–12 hours
5 oz/150 g flaxseeds, soaked 8–12 hours
20 drops stevia or 2 tsp stevia powder
1 tsp cinnamon
4 oz/120 g raisins

Soak the nuts and seeds overnight in 32 fl oz (1 liter) of water. Put them in the blender with the stevia and cinnamon, and blend until there are no seeds discernable in the mix. Stir in the raisins by hand. Spread onto dehydrator trays, and dry for 12 hours. Slice, turn, and dry for 2–4 more hours.

These were our favorites for a long while. I didn't know what to call them until Ethan asked for one of those "lovely biscuits" one day and the name stuck.

HOT CROSS BUNS

Blender, dehydrator
10 minutes (8–12 hours presoaking, 18 hours dehydrating)
Makes 24 buns

*Hot cross buns are one of those seasonal treats it's often hard to let
go of. The aromatic spices, the chewy dried fruit, the doughy bun. . . .
For a couple of years after the family had given up wheat entirely,
I compromised and bought a wheat-free soda bread dough mix.
I just added in some spices and raisins and made a giant wheat-free
hot cross bun. But once the boys had really stopped eating cooked
altogether, I had to come up with a raw version. Here it is!*

10 oz/300 g oats, presoaked 8–12 hours

4 tbsp agave nectar

4 tbsp olive oil

2 tbsp mixed spice

8 fl oz/250 ml water

7 oz/200 g mixed raisins

2 tbsp yacon syrup or molasses

2 tbsp tahini

Soak your oats overnight. You can use oat groats or rolled oats, whichever
you prefer. Put the oats, agave, olive oil, mixed spice, and water in the
blender, and blend to a thick batter. Stir in the raisins by hand. Using a teaspoon, put dollops of the mixture on the dehydrator tray, nice and fat, like
little buns. They should ideally be about $^3/_4$ inch high, and $2^1/_2$ inches in
diameter. Dry for 18 hours. When they're done, mix up the molasses and
tahini with a spoon or two of water so it is not too stiff to spread, and not so
runny that it won't stick. Using a teaspoon, you should be able to drizzle a
cross on top of the buns.

*Yacon syrup is available from the online raw food stores.
It is a sugar-free sweetener made from a Peruvian root
vegetable, which tastes similar to barley malt syrup
but has no impact on the blood sugar.*

Coconut Carob Cookies

Blender, food processor, dehydrator

10 minutes (12 hours dehydrating)

Makes about 20 cookies

These are very rich—save as treats!

8 oz/250 g pitted dates

2 bananas, peeled and chopped

2 oz/60 g carob powder

9 oz/270 g fresh coconut

Blend dates, banana, and carob together to a puree. Chop the coconut into small pieces, and grate it in the food processor so you have small chunks no bigger than raisins. Stir into the carob mix by hand. Put spoonfuls of the mixture onto the dehydrator trays, flattening down so they are not too thick—ideally about $1/2$ inch. Dry for 12 hours.

If you're a raw chocoholic, substitute the carob
for raw chocolate powder.

Apple Cashew Cookies

Blender, dehydrator

5 minutes (8–12 hours presoaking, 18 hours dehydrating)

Makes about 20 cookies

These are really great—tasty, and so quick to make. So quick to eat too;
whenever we make a batch of these they're gone in minutes.

4 oz/120 g cashews, presoaked 8–12 hours

1 lb/500 g apples

4 oz/120 g raisins

Presoak the cashews. If you forget, you can just grind them up and add them to the mix; it will still work fine. Chop the apples into pieces that are a manageable size for your blender. Blend the apples and cashews together, and once you've got a puree, with no bits of nut remaining, stir in the raisins by hand. Put spoonfuls on your dehydrator tray, about $\frac{1}{2}$ inch high. Dry for 12 hours, flip, and dry for another 6 hours.

Drinking fresh-pressed apple juice helps reduce the risk of kidney stones. A popular cleansing technique is to fast for three days on apple juice, which softens the stones, then to drink a mix of olive oil and lemon juice to flush the stones out. Not exactly delicious, but it works.

Chocolate Brownies

Blender, dehydrator

10 minutes (8–12 hours presoaking, 18 hours dehydrating)

Makes 16 brownies

This has to be the king of my mainstay recipes! Using the wondrous cacao bean, these taste so good, as well as giving you such a hit of pure cacao magic.

10 oz/300 g oats, soaked 8–12 hours

4 oz/120 g ground cacao

4 oz/120 g pitted fresh dates
(or 4 tbsp agave syrup and 4 fl oz/125 ml water)

4 fl oz/125 ml olive oil

1 tbsp maca powder (optional, for an extra buzz)

2 tbsp carob powder

4 tbsp carob chips (not raw, optional)

Presoak your oats. You can use rolled oats or groats, whichever you prefer. Put all the ingredients apart from the carob chips in the blender, and process to a thick puree. Stir in the carob chips or raisins if you prefer, by hand. Spoon the mixture onto a dehydrating tray, about $\frac{1}{2}$ inch thick. Form into a square shape. Dry for 12 hours and then score into 16 squares (4 by 4). Turn and dry for a further 6 hours. Stored in an airtight container in the fridge, they will keep for a couple of weeks.

These make a great mid-morning snack, as the oats (a slow-release carbohydrate) stabilize blood sugar levels for the day and the cacao gives you a boost to help you breeze through to lunch.

Carrot Cakes

Blender, dehydrator

10 minutes (12 hours dehydrating)

Makes 12 cakes

The ground flaxseeds give these a kind of yeasty taste that, along with the spices and dried fruit, makes them just like little buns.

5 oz/150 g ground flaxseeds

1 apple

4 carrots

1 tbsp mixed spice

2 tbsp raisins

Grind the flaxseeds in a coffee grinder or high-powered blender. Chop and core the apple; top and tail the carrots. Chop them into blender-friendly size pieces, pop them in, and puree them. Add the ground flaxseeds and mixed spice and puree again. Stir in the raisins by hand. You should have a fairly firm mixture. Shape it into patties between the palms of your hands, getting them as thin as you can without them falling apart. You should have about a dozen little cakes. Spread on a drying tray and dry for 6 hours, turn over, and dry for another 6 hours.

*Carrots were the first vegetable to be canned,
in the early nineteenth century.*

FLAPJACKS

Blender, dehydrator

10 minutes (8–12 hours soaking, 18 hours dehydrating)

Makes 20 flapjacks

This is a slight variation on an old favorite.

10 oz/300 g oats, soaked 8–12 hours

4 tbsp agave nectar

4 tbsp olive oil

4 tbsp water

4 oz/120 g raisins

Put everything except for the raisins in the blender. Blend to an oatmeal (you can eat it like this for breakfast if you want!). Stir in the raisins by hand. Spread onto a drying tray, about an inch thick. Dry for 12 hours, then score into squares, 4 by 5, or possibly 5 by 5 if you want to make little ones. Flip over, and dry for a further 6 hours. Store in an airtight container, and keep for up to two weeks.

Variations:

Honestly, we make these every week and we never get bored of them. Try blending in

- 2 tbsp carob powder
- 2 tbsp goji berries, soaked 1–2 hours
- 2 tbsp bee pollen
- 2 tbsp maca powder
- 2 tbsp fresh dates instead of agave
- 1 tbsp cinnamon, or mixed spice
- 1 inch fresh root ginger
- 10 drops orange oil

CANDY

Here are some little nibbles that should be enough to persuade even the most reluctant among you that raw food isn't boring and bland. Whip these out to impress guests and children on birthdays, at Christmas—in fact, at every available opportunity! These are sweets that you can eat without worrying about ruining your appetite—they have more nutrition in them than a "proper meal" like pasta and jarred sauce or a frozen dinner.

SPECIAL SWEETIES

Gear juicer or food processor

30 minutes

Makes about 20 pieces

Pine nuts and macadamias make a gorgeously decadent combination, rich and luxurious and positively naughty! If your budget won't stretch to both, you could substitute hulled sesame seeds for one or the other.

4 oz/120 g pine nuts

4 oz/120 g macadamia nuts

4 oz/120 g pitted fresh dates

Pinch sea salt

1 tbsp agave nectar

3 oz/90 g carob powder

There are two ways of making these. The best way is to feed them through a gear juicer with the blank plate on, nuts first, then dates. Add a pinch of sea salt to the mixing bowl, and using a spoon or your hands mix everything together. If you don't have a gear juicer, you can grind the nuts first, and then put everything together in the food processor. You don't get as smooth a candy, but it still works. Take the mixture and form into walnut-sized balls. Store in the fridge—will keep for a few weeks.

For Valentine's Day, or as a gift for a loved one, shape the candy mix into hearts, about ¹/₂ inch thick and 1¹/₂ inches long; then pour some melted raw chocolate or carob over the top for icing.

GREEN LEATHERS

Blender, dehydrator

5 minutes (12 hours dehydrating)

Makes 4 leathers

How many children do you know that will eat kale gladly? As a matter of fact, not many adults like kale either. In my quest to get greens in my boys, I came up with these. Despite each one containing a decent serving of kale, the end result just tastes like a sweet treat.

4 apples

1 lb/500 g kale

Chop the apples, remove the cores. Put the apple pieces in the blender, and blend to a puree. Then prepare the kale: discard any large stems, chop into little bits, and add to the apple puree. Puree until you have no bits left, and the mix is a gorgeous deep green. Spread onto a dehydrator tray and dry for 12 hours, until it will peel smoothly off the tray. Roll up, and then slice them into two across the middle. Store in an airtight container in a cool place. These leathers will keep for up to a month.

This was inspired by a yummy raw snack bar called the ReBar, which tastes just like a normal fruit bar but contains kale, broccoli, spinach, even wheatgrass!

SALAD BAR

Blender, dehydrator

5 minutes (12 hours dehydrating)

Makes 4 bars

Similar to the previous recipe, this is a salad in a snack bar.
Don't tell your children it's got vegetables in it and they'll never know!

1 apple

2 sticks celery

4 leaves lettuce

1 tomato

$\frac{1}{4}$ cucumber

Prepare all the ingredients for the blender by chopping into manageable chunks. Discard the apple core. If you're using leafy celery, remove the leaves: they are health giving but bitter and will overpower the flavor of the bar. Toss everything in the blender, and whiz it up to a liquid. Have a taste: if it's not sweet enough for you, add an extra apple. Spread onto two drying trays, and dry for 12 hours. When they're pliable, not at all soggy (underdone) or crisp (overdone), they're ready. Take them out, roll them up, and slice them into two across the middle. Store in an airtight container in the fridge. The bars will keep for up to a month.

Celery is rich in sodium, containing about 35 mg in each stalk.
So if you are craving salt, try adding extra celery to your
food and see if that helps lessen your cravings.

JAM

Blender

5 minutes (4–8 hours soaking)

Makes 2 jars

This jam is good for spreading on crackers or Essene (sprouted) bread.
It tastes just like those sugar-free fruit jams you can buy,
and is so quick and easy to make.

2 oz/60 g prunes, soaked 4–8 hours

3 apples

1 lemon, juiced

Soak the prunes in advance. Core and chop the apples, and put the pieces in the blender. Blend until you have a puree. Add the prunes and lemon juice, and puree again. Stored in jars in the fridge, the jam will keep for about five days.

> *Variation:* replace the prunes with unsulfured dried apricots for apricot jam.

RAW CHOCOLATE

Food grinder, food processor

30 minutes

Makes 20 pieces (or 1 if you're my ex-husband)

*The cacao bean is what all chocolate is made from. The raw bean is a
relative newcomer to the raw food scene. It's so good, I wouldn't be
surprised if they tried to make it illegal. I can't get enough of it—
it makes me feel happier, full of energy, more productive, less hungry—
life is a breeze! For a decadent, delectable sweet try this truffle recipe.*

4 oz/120 g cacao beans or nibs

4 oz/120 g sesame seeds

1 vanilla pod

4 oz/120 g pitted fresh dates

Grind up the cacao, sesame seeds, and vanilla in a food grinder or high-powered blender. Mash the dates up in the food processor. We only use 4 oz (120 g) dates, which makes a very deep chocolatey truffle, a bit like plain chocolate. If you have a sweet tooth, you may want to add more dates or a tablespoon of agave nectar. Add the vanilla, seeds, and cacao to the food processor and turn until the mixture balls up. Break into walnut-sized pieces and form into small balls. If the chocolates are for a gift or a party, coat them in desiccated coconut for a professional finish. Alternatively, you can just leave the mix in one big lump and eat huge chunks like my ex-husband does. Whichever way, it needs to be stored in the fridge.

*There are dozens of raw chocolate bars on the market today.
If your local health food store doesn't stock them, ask them to
get some in. Once people get into the raw chocolate habit,
invariably they don't want to go back to the cooked stuff.
Raw Living was the first company to retail raw
chocolate bars in the United Kingdom.*

MACA BALLS

No equipment needed

10 minutes

Makes 16 balls

*Maca is a fantastic super food, full of protein and minerals
and very energizing. Its flavor goes very well with carob.
Have one (or two) of these mid-morning or late afternoon
when you're starting to flag, to perk you up.*

2 heaped tbsp maca powder

2 oz/60 g carob powder

8 oz/250 g tahini

2 tbsp agave

Put all the ingredients in a mixing bowl, and combine with a spoon. Roll into walnut-sized balls—makes about 16. Stored in an airtight container in the fridge, they should keep for weeks.

*The maca plant grows at higher altitudes than any other plant
in the world. It can also withstand extremes of temperature—
intense heat and biting cold. So it provides us with that energy
of endurance, of being able to battle through life no matter
how high the mountain or how fierce the storm!*

SUPER SWEETIES

Gear juicer or food grinder, food processor

20 minutes

Makes 25–30 truffles

These have got everything going on in them. They are wonderful for parties to get everyone in a lively festive spirit. What's more, they're so packed with vitamins and minerals, you could virtually live on them.

8 oz/250 g cacao nibs

3 oz/90 g goji berries

2 tbsp maca powder

2 tbsp bee pollen granules

1 tbsp Klamath Lake blue-green algae powder

2 tbsp agave syrup

2 oz/60 g carob powder

Pinch crystal or sea salt

If you have a gear juicer, put the cacao and goji berries through with the blank plate on. If not, grind the cacao in a grinder, and mash the gojis separately in the food processor. Then put all the ingredients together in the food processor, and keep it turning until the mixture balls up. If it doesn't start sticking, add a few drops of water to help it along. Once you've got a solid mass, break off walnut-sized pieces and shape into balls. Stored in an airtight container in the fridge, they should keep for up to a month.

Our favorite type of blue-green algae is called Crystal Manna. It comes as flakes and looks just like green glitter— it has to be seen to be believed. We sprinkle it on our dinner or add it to our chocolate.

GUEST RECIPES

Raw is getting more and more popular by the day, which is fantastic. But the number of people who have been doing it a long time is actually quite small. Ten years ago it was very hard to sustain the diet when there was so little information and support around, and many people who believed that this way of eating was beneficial found they couldn't integrate it into their existing lifestyles, or didn't have the knowledge to make it work for them. That's why those people who have stuck at it over the years really deserve recognition and support. They are pioneers, making mistakes and learning the hard way, so they can share their lessons with you. Here is a selection of recipes by some of my very favorite raw fooders in the UK. Dig in!

A Different Kind of Recipe for Salad Success

Steve Charter

Steve is a long-term raw foodist who has been actively promoting the benefits of the diet for well over a decade. He comes from a permaculture background and works hard to get raw foods recognized as an integral part of sustainable living.

Take the seeds of a wide range of perennial and self-seeding salad plants—these might be arugula, lettuces, endive, different kales, tomatoes, perennial spinach, chard, oriental salad greens such as Mitsuna or mustard greens, chicory, celery, lovage, and so on—and add a few seeds of edible flowers such as nasturtiums, mallow, and calendula. Sprinkle these lightly in appropriate parts of the garden, in large pots, or in window boxes. Add water. Add more water according to climatic needs on the days following the day of sowing and then as needed during the growth of the plants. Leave in the sun for two to four months, and then harvest and eat with some of the other fabulous recipes detailed in this book . . .

Permaculture means permanent agriculture. It is a methodology of sustainable living that seeks to work in harmony with nature and follow the patterns of ecology.

Manhattan Sub-Cumber Sandwich

Joel "Cosmic CacaoBoy" Gazdar

*Joel has been pioneering the evolution of raw foods toward
"SuperLifeFood" since 2000. He currently writes for the rawinspirations
e-zine. He makes the best food I have ever eaten. Ever.*

1 cucumber (wider girth preferable)

2 oz/60 g freshly ground pumpkin seeds and/or hemp seeds

1 tsp (virgin, preferably stone-crushed) olive oil or raw tahini

1 tsp unpasteurized apple cider vinegar or lemon juice

1 clove fresh garlic

1 sprig fresh dill weed/cilantro/basil

Sprinkle of caraway seed

1 tsp raw (preferably wildflower/unfiltered) honey or dried
(unsulfured) apricots

1 tsp unrefined sea salt

Remove the tip from a cucumber (ridged or plain), preferably not too cold.
Hollow out with appropriate diameter copper pipe, chopstick, or type of
spoon used to scoop marrow out of bone (by leaving one end of the
cucumber sealed you lessen the chances of squirting the filling every-
where). Save the juicy seedy core for salad or a dressing. To make the filling, take all the other ingredients and either mix in a bowl, grind in a
blender, or mash in a mortar and pestle. Stuff the length of the cuke till
full, and allow up to an hour for marinade to diffuse inside. Enjoy!

*Cucumber is thought to derive from "cowcumber," because at
one time they were thought to be fit only for feeding to cows!
Cucumber skins are high in silica. Silica (sand) is known
as the beauty mineral, and is beneficial for elasticity
of tissues and whole-brain functioning.*

MUSHROOM AND SEAWEED SAUCE

Rob Hull

*Rob is a good friend based in London who works full-time promoting
raw foods through the Funky Raw website and magazine.*

1 oz/30 g sea spaghetti seaweed, soaked for about 20 minutes

3 oz/90 g mushrooms

1 medium avocado

Presoak the sea spaghetti. Chop the mushrooms and avocado and place in a blender with the sea spaghetti and the soak water, and blend. This makes quite a rich sauce to serve with salad.

*Funky Raw was founded in 2004 by Tish Clifford, a long-term
raw fooder and mother of two children, in order to provide
a voice for the raw food movement in the United Kingdom,
particularly those seeking to use raw foods as a vehicle
for personal development and global change.*

SUPER FOOD "COOKIE DOUGH" BALLS

Jess Michael

*Princess Jess is a raw food superstar in the making. Be sure to check her
out if you want some inspiring yet down-to-earth raw wisdom. Jess is
the founder of Total Raw Food (see www.totalrawfood.com).*

13 oz/390 g of your favorite nuts (cashew and almond
work well together), soaked for at least $1/_2$ hour

$1/_3$ cup of coconut butter

4 oz/120 g raisins

2 oz/60 g fresh, juicy dates

3 tsp cinnamon

Seeds from 1 vanilla pod

$1/_2$ tsp Atlantic/Himalayan rock salt (optional)

2 oz/60 g goji berries (optional, yet highly recommended!)

4 tbsp raw chocolate powder/ground-down raw cacao nibs

3 tbsp agave nectar (optional, as the mixture might be sweet enough
for you already!)

Presoak the nuts. If your coconut butter is solid, melt it down into liquid
over a low heat. Add all the ingredients to your food processor and mix until
a doughlike texture occurs. Taste your creation, to check for sweetness and
texture. You might want to add the agave, if it's not sweet enough, or some
more coconut butter if you want it to be more blended. Time to get messy!
Get a good spoonful of "cookie dough" at a time and roll it into a ball in the
palms of your hands. Refrigerate or eat right away . . . you choose!

I usually double or triple the batches of these great cookie dough balls,
as they just never seem to stick around for too long! If you put them in the
fridge for a few hours afterward, they go solid, which makes for the best-
ever travel snack!

*Jess suffered from chronic fatigue syndrome when she was
younger and used the raw food diet to help rid herself of
this debilitating condition. Now she runs her own business,
puts on popular workshops, and even runs marathons!*

GOLDEN CHERRY CREAM PIE

Holly Paige

Holly is a gorgeous and outspoken figure on the raw food circuit. If she's doing an event, you're never quite sure what to expect, but you know it's going to be enlivening and enriching.

Pastry

3 oz/90 g almonds, soaked

3 oz/90 g hazelnuts/filberts, soaked and dehydrated if possible

5 dates, fresh if possible

5 prunes

1 banana

1 oz/30 g pitted dried cherries, or goji berries if not available

Handful cacao nibs

Topping

7 fl oz/200 ml hemp milk made with 3 oz/90 g hemp seeds
and juice of 2 oranges and extra water as necessary

A few pieces orange peel/zest

2 dried figs

$\frac{1}{2}$ banana

2 oz/60 g macadamia nuts

1 oz/30 g goji berries

Handful fresh cherries

Sprinkling raw chocolate powder

Process all the pastry ingredients except the cacao nibs together until smooth. Mix in the nibs and form the pastry base on a plate. Blend the topping ingredients together until smooth, and fill the pie. It will set in a few minutes. Sprinkle the raw chocolate powder on the top and decorate with halved cherries.

Holly is a big fan of raw dairy produce for her growing children. Most raw fooders are vegan, but Holly and others find raw dairy such as unpasteurized goat's cheese and yogurt an essential part of the road to optimum health.

MELOMACAROUNA: "HONEY" CAKES

Gina Panayi

Gina is unique in approaching raw foods from a Greek culinary perspective. She takes traditional Greek dishes and makes raw adaptations.

4 medjool dates

8 fl oz/250 ml agave syrup

8 fl oz/250 ml fresh orange juice

2 tbsp orange rind/zest

15 oz/450 g ground almonds, soaked overnight

3 oz/90 g ground golden flaxseeds

2 tsp cinnamon

1 tsp Celtic sea salt

Crushed walnuts for decorating

Put the dates through the juicer and then place in the blender with the agave syrup, orange juice, and zest. Blend together until all the ingredients are well mixed. Drain and rinse the almonds and feed through the juicer with the blank plate. Place in the food processor with the ground flaxseed, cinnamon, and salt and very briefly pulsate. Pour some of the liquid from the blender into the food processor and process while adding more liquid a little at a time until it all starts to bind and the mixture is evenly mixed together. Take small pieces of the mixture with your hands and form into oval cookie shapes. Place the cakes onto a dehydrator tray. Crush or lightly grind the walnuts and sprinkle on top of the cakes and place in the dehydrator on 145°F for about 3 hours and then at 115°F for another 2 hours. These cakes should be slightly crispy on the outside but soft and moist on the inside. Makes approximately 20 cakes.

Medjool dates are probably the most popular among raw fooders; plump and tender, one is a whole meal in itself. There are many other varieties available, especially in Middle Eastern grocers. Look for the yellow ones on the vine— they are usually hard, but take them home and let them ripen and they taste divine.

TOBY ROAMED

Shazzie

Shazzie is one of the most beautiful beings I have ever encountered: everything she does comes from the heart and she is doing amazing work to increase the amount of love and joy in people's lives. Shazzie, managing director of Rawcreation Ltd., has been an ethical vegan since 1997 and a raw foodist since 2000, has written three books, and runs the website www.shazzie.com. We don't fight over the crown to be the United Kingdom's most popular raw food writer and promoter; we like to get together and have a giggle over the whole thing instead.

4 oz/120 g cacao nibs

4 oz/120 g cashew nuts

7 oz/200 g cacao butter

2 oz/60 g raw carob powder

4 tbsp raw agave nectar

1 tsp Blue Manna powder

1 tsp maca

2$\frac{1}{2}$ tbsp coconut oil

Grind the cacao nibs into a fine powder. Grind the cashew nuts into a fine powder. Grate the white cacao butter and add to a bowl. Pour some warm water into another bowl and sit the bowl with the butter into this bowl. Don't get water into your cacao butter. Wait until the butter has melted, and then add the other ingredients. Stir very well and then pour it into any pretty molds.

Oooh, this is so much like that triangular Swiss chocolate that we all love. Er, except this one's got masses of brain food in it.

LOTUS, NORI, AND RED WINE SALAD

Ysanne Spevack

One of my oldest and dearest friends, Ysanne is a hugely talented food writer with a passion for organics, who now lives in LA.. She has written thirteen books on organic food and organic living and is editor of www.organicfood.co.uk. She is also a founding consultant editor of Organic *magazine in the United Kingdom.*

2 tbsp red wine

2 tbsp olive oil

1 tbsp tahini

1 tbsp black sesame seeds

4 oz/120 g rehydrated dried lotus root

2 big sheets of nori, torn into $\frac{1}{2}$ inch squares

Shake the wine and oil together in a small container to form a dressing. Add the tahini and mix in with a fork, squashing any lumps to blend it in. Then mix in the seeds, and pour the dressing over the lotus root. Leave to marinate for at least 20 minutes before serving. Just before the salad is eaten, sprinkle on the nori.

This rich and decadent salad is a great winter warmer, due to the wine. It's a salad you can pull out of nowhere, as it's made entirely from ingredients you can keep in your storage cupboard. It's so strongly flavored; I recommend you eat it as a starter rather than a side dish. Invented in California, I was inspired by the mix of Japanese sushi culture found there alongside the local penchant for fine Napa Valley wines. This is a truly eccentrically English take on the Californian culinary scene. And yes, wine is raw!

Lotus root is very nutritious and popular in both Chinese and Indian cuisine. The lotus flower is a symbol of divine beauty in Hindu and Buddhist cultures.

SEDUCTIVELY SQUISHED SALAD

Angela Stokes

Angela's amazing weight-loss story is an inspiration to thousands. Born and bred in South England, these days Gela is to be found traveling the globe, sharing her adventures with like-minded souls and recording the events on her popular website, www.rawreform.com.

Head of 1 romaine lettuce sliced into thin strips,
or a few good handfuls of young salad greens

Small bunch of cilantro, chopped very finely

$\frac{1}{2}$ cucumber, grated

2 carrots, grated

$\frac{1}{2}$ red bell pepper, sliced into small chunks

Handful of dulse, shredded small

1 lemon or lime, juiced

1 tsp kelp powder, or pinch of Himalayan sea salt, to taste

Flesh of 1 avocado, in rough pieces

Any other "garnishes" of choice—for example,
chopped chives, fresh sprouts, nuts, and so on

Combine all of the ingredients in a big bowl. Then with your hand squish the whole mixture together until it is all evenly distributed and the avocado has spread out through all the other ingredients, like a dressing. I love this method because it removes the need for any other salad dressing, like heavy oils, and is so easy to prepare with a minimum amount of fuss or equipment. I call this "seductively squished salad" as you then get to lick the remaining ingredients from your hand after the squishing, if you so desire. Makes enough for one, or two, depending on how hungry (and friendly) you are! This is my current favorite salad, which I tend to prepare around the middle of the day to tank me up on raw nutrition for the rest of the day.

In 2007, Gela embarked on a ninety-two-day juice feast. The idea of this is not that you fast, but that by consuming only liquids you can still get an abundance of nutrients and calories, thus helping your body to detoxify while ensuring it gets plenty of nourishment.

RICH "NO" CHOCOLATE MOUSSE

Jill Swyers

*Jill is a Hippocrates Health educator, and a much-loved and respected
member of the raw foods community. She divides her time
between London, Portugal, and Florida, holding raw
workshops, retreats, and trainings.*

5 oz/150 g walnuts, soaked in water overnight

3 oz/90 g pine nuts, soaked in water overnight

7 oz/200 g dates, soaked in water to just cover dates

3 oz/90 g carob powder

$\frac{1}{2}$ soft avocado (if available)

$\frac{1}{2}$ lemon, freshly juiced

Throw away water from nuts and rinse. Process walnuts and pine nuts in
food processor. Add dates. Add carob powder, avocado, and lemon. Place
in dish. Leave in refrigerator for 2 hours or overnight. Decorate with raspberries, strawberries, or edible flowers—enjoy.

*At Hippocrates Health Institute they are big advocates
of indoor greens. These are seed trays planted with seeds
that are allowed to sprout and germinate and are usually
consumed when they are a week or two old. As well as the
more commonly known barleygrass and wheatgrass,
they also use buckwheat, sunflower, and pea greens.*

Recommended Reading

Raw Classics

The Sunfood Diet Success System or anything else by David Wolfe

Rainbow Green Live-Food Cuisine or anything else by Gabriel Cousens

Raw by Juliano, the original gourmet raw recipe book

The Politics of Food

Fast Food Nation by Eric Schlosser

Not on the Label and *Eat Your Heart Out* by Felicity Lawrence

Shopped by Joanna Blythman

Educational Websites

www.thebestdayever.com
David Wolfe's amazing website on raw foods and cutting-edge nutrition

www.naturalnews.com
Independent news on natural health, nutrition, and more from Mike
Adams and team

www.whfoods.com
The World's Healthiest Foods, comprehensive nutritional information
from George Mateljan

Index

About the Author

Kate Wood is the most experienced raw food promoter in the United Kingdom. She has been following a raw diet since 1993, and is raising a family of three boys on a predominantly raw diet. She is the author of *Eat Smart, Eat Raw*, the UK's best selling raw food recipe book; published originally by Grub Street in 2002. Her third book, *Raw Magic*, a groundbreaking book of superfood recipes—another UK first—was published by Rawcreation in 2008, to rave reviews.

She is a managing director of the Raw Living website, which offers advice and information on the raw diet, as well as an online shop. She is also the proud parent of the Raw Living range of chocolate bars and cakes. For three years, she was the editor of *Get Fresh* magazine, the world's most popular raw food magazine. She currently divides her time between being with her children and doing private consultations. She has two books out in 2009, *Ecstatic Beings* (co-authored with Shazzie) about the joy and bliss that results from living a holistic, tuned-in life, and *88-the Untold Story of a Revolution* (about the original London acid house scene). She is also developing a fledgling music career.

Kate has been featured in most of the UK's national press including *The Independent, The Guardian, The Sunday Times, The Daily Express, Metro, Vogue, Marie Claire, Cosmopolitan, Red, Zest, Closer, Reveal, The Green Parent, Lifescape, Juno, Get Fresh,* and *Funky Raw.* She has made a number of national media appearances including BBC TV and radio, ITV, Channel 4, Passion for the Planet digital radio, and Radio Reverb. She has spoken at numerous festivals and events around the country, primarily on raw foods, but also on superfoods and on natural parenting.

Kate is driven by a passionate desire for change in this world. Everything she does is fueled by her vision of humanity living together in peace and unity, and restoring our mother earth to a garden paradise. She believes raw foods and superfoods are an important tool in unlocking our inner potential and empowering ourselves as individuals to create the revolution that is so urgently needed at this time.